"It's so difficult to explain depression to someone
who's never been there,
because it's not just sadness."

J.K. Rowling

ISBN 978-0-6452517-1-5

Also available as e-book ISBN 978-0-6452517-0-8

www.blackdogsherbal.com

The beautiful images are attributed to the photographers.

Cover image by StockSnap from Pixabay.

Black Dog's Herbal

a conversation to de-puzzle depression

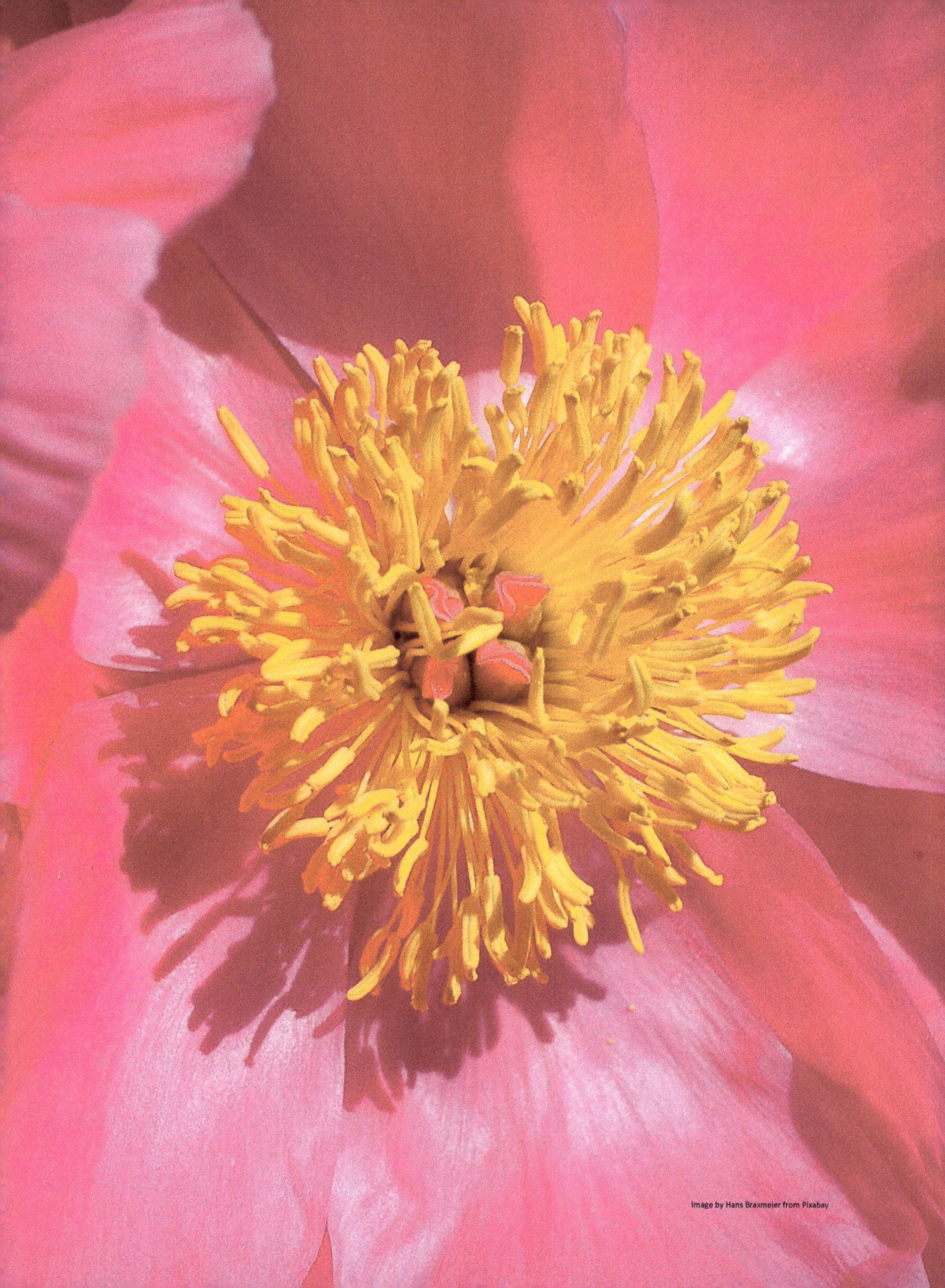

Image by Hans Braxmeier from Pixabay

Peony - Paeonia lactiflora

Peony is native to Central Asia, with a natural range from Tibet across central China and limited by Siberia. It has been used in Chinese medicine for thousands of years, and the flowers are enormously esteemed in Asia in much the same way roses are in Europe. It has been recorded in Chinese literature as far back as 3,900 years ago. Today, the plant can be found all over the world due to the desire to have its beauty in gardens and parks. Traditionally, the white roots of the Peony are thought to be the best part of the plant for medicinal use. However, numerous cultivars have been created with different colours and flower structure, and it may be assumed that they all contain similar properties to the primary plant source of the medicine being Paeonia lactiflora. Many intensive farms are growing, harvesting, and selling its medicinal roots, which are called 'shaoyao' in China. However, debates are ongoing as to the regions that have the best therapeutic material.

The main compound found in Peony is paeoniflorin and it has been studied in isolation from the rest of the chemical compounds in the plant. In research from Hong Kong in 2013 it was found that paeoniflorin increased serotonin levels and that it was comparable to the standard antidepressant drug imipramine. Doses of 40 mg/kg body weight of Paeoniflorin had the best results in the testing. It should however be noted that this was one of many compounds found within the plant.

Another study (2017), this time from mainland China, compared the root extract to the standard drug fluoxetine. In this study it was found that giving an oral dose of 600 mg/kg body weight had better results than the standard medication. However, the extract took approximately 2 weeks to achieve this. Such a delay is not uncommon in standard drugs and therefore should pose no great challenge in its use as the side effects are far less than the standard antidepressant drugs.

The herb has also been found to protect the neurons of the brain, especially in the hippocampus region. This neuroprotective action of the herb is in addition to the increase of serotonin. As a result, many other trials have been undertaken to assess the potential of Paeonia extract in the treatment of dementia and other neurological diseases of the aged and young alike.

In China the traditional uses of the plant have also focused on women's issues such as dysmenorrhea (painful period cramps) and also as a liver tonic. In saying, this herb for depression may be a preferred choice for women even though men will have the same antidepressant results.

It is comforting to know that Paeonia lactiflora has been included in the World Health Organisation's (WHO) list of essential medicines and is easily found in the herbal monographs on their website.

[1] F. Qiu, X. Zhong, Q. Mao, and Z. Huang, "The antidepressant-like effects of paeoniflorin in mouse models," Exp. Ther. Med., vol. 5, no. 4, pp. 1113–1116, 2013.

[2] X. hui Yu et al., "Anti-depressant effect of Paeonia lactiflora pall extract in rats," Trop. J. Pharm. Res., vol. 16, no. 3, pp. 577–580, 2017.

[3] X. Zhong, G. Li, F. Qiu, and Z. Huang, "Paeoniflorin ameliorates chronic stress-induced depression-like behaviours and neuronal damages in rats via activation of the ERK-CREB pathway," Front. Psychiatry, vol. 10, no. JAN, pp. 1–8, 2019.

[4] D. P. Sinica, M. Parle, and K. Sharma, "Pelagia Research Library Medicinal plants possessing anxiolytic activity: A brief review," vol. 6, no. 5, pp. 1–7, 2015.

Preface

If you lecture, force advice, impose your opinion, dismiss, cajole, coax, flatter or compel a person who is suffering from depression, then in all likelihood your efforts will fail. You may think for a while that you have succeeded in alleviating their depression, yet all you might have done is fallen for an easy smile, a sly joke, and a statement declaring that "everything is fine", whilst all the while the depression continues.

Depression is a conversation, a journey better shared if possible. Depression is personal evolution through sadness, loneliness, and pain. This book started as a simple reference resource for antidepressant and anti-anxiety herbs, yet the common mistake was quickly recognized that depression is a multifaceted condition requiring a multipronged management system. A simple herb or drug simply will not cut it. A conversation is needed. So now the stunning herbs are surrounded by part of that conversation within this book.

Interesting to note that herbs have been around for a long, long, time and during their history they have been associated with witches who would have been the poster girls for depression as they lived alone under thatched roofs at the edges of villages or towns, talking to black cats. We do not know of their loneliness or sadness as they knew a thing or two about the best herbs to use to take your mind off troubles and woes. This book is not about witches, thatched cottages and black cats. We are talking about depression, black dogs and herbs that have been used throughout history, and that have now been to sterile clinical laboratories where serious men and women in white lab coats have tested them. The herbs not the witches.

It may come as a surprise to you, but when we think about it, the world would be a much better place if more people were depressed! A depressed person is seeking answers and most of these answers deal with making life meaningful. A depressed person does not care about money or mansions by the sea, as these have enough suicides on their floors. A depressed person cares about the future and the lack of meaning in it. Within depression's embrace, a person will dream of a better world, not an empty love affair. Only when someone has hit rock bottom do they gain insight and comprehension into another person's pain and suffering, and only then will they be equipped to help.

Depression has given the world breath-taking art and music.

Depression has written words of the deepest insight and beauty.

Depression has solved some of the greatest mysteries of science.

Depression grabs a person and removes the sunglasses of ignorance, forcing them to look directly into the sun of truth. Uncomfortable. Unyielding. Unforgiving.

With far less side effects and significantly less cost, herbs and their use are able to give a feeling of control to an otherwise out of control condition.

For the past several decades science and therapists have tried to label depression as a disease and illness, yet it has defied their attempts at its containment, resulting in vast numbers of populations disappearing into it, a black hole. It can be an uncomfortable space if there is no way out. Understanding your depression leads to the ability to control it, to a way out.

So, what is depression? Perhaps we may never really know. But for me, in my bitter romance with the grey lover, I have come to appreciate my depression. I have found my interpretation of it, just as one artist will interpret a sunrise completely different from all others. For me depression is an intellectual evolution. A coming of age. Depression I find is a poor term to describe the growth of awareness unasked for. Uncalled for. But undeniable and critical for our species to survive. Depression is both a curse and a gift.

As with all things in life the right perspective is crucial. Sitting on a mountain top the views are vast and limitless whilst down in the valleys they are short and restricted.

The same applies to depression as we navigate the highs and lows of its dark ocean waves. Having a mascot dog, imaginary or real makes no difference as depression is a construct of our own minds. Taking a mascot dog on imaginary or real walks in this grey world is to help us colour our minds differently. In essence, the wisdom of Winston Churchill and his black dog is now taken literally.

Yet, the symbolism of the black dog, corresponds to more cultures.

In Caucasian culture the colour black not only represents loss, evil and depression but also mystery, sophistication, elegance and the unknown. The link of colour to the dog whose representations range from loyalty, truthfulness to self, vigilance, and protection offers a very apt and fitting mascot for our journey in the grey realm.

In China the dog is a revered animal and one of the Chinese zodiac symbols. The dog represents both good and bad, but it is best known to avert disasters and chase away demons and monsters. The colour black in China is the colour of water, and whilst the colour symbolises bad fortune, destruction, evil, profundity, sadness and suffering, black is also the colour for heaven, delving into depth, knowledge, stability, and power.

In the Aztec and Mayan cultures dogs were sacred and served their master to ward off evil spirits in even after death.

This marriage of colour with the dog is intriguing. I myself approach depression from the perspective of wonder, mystery and adventure, and this seems to me an adequate start to connect to this companion.

Table of Content

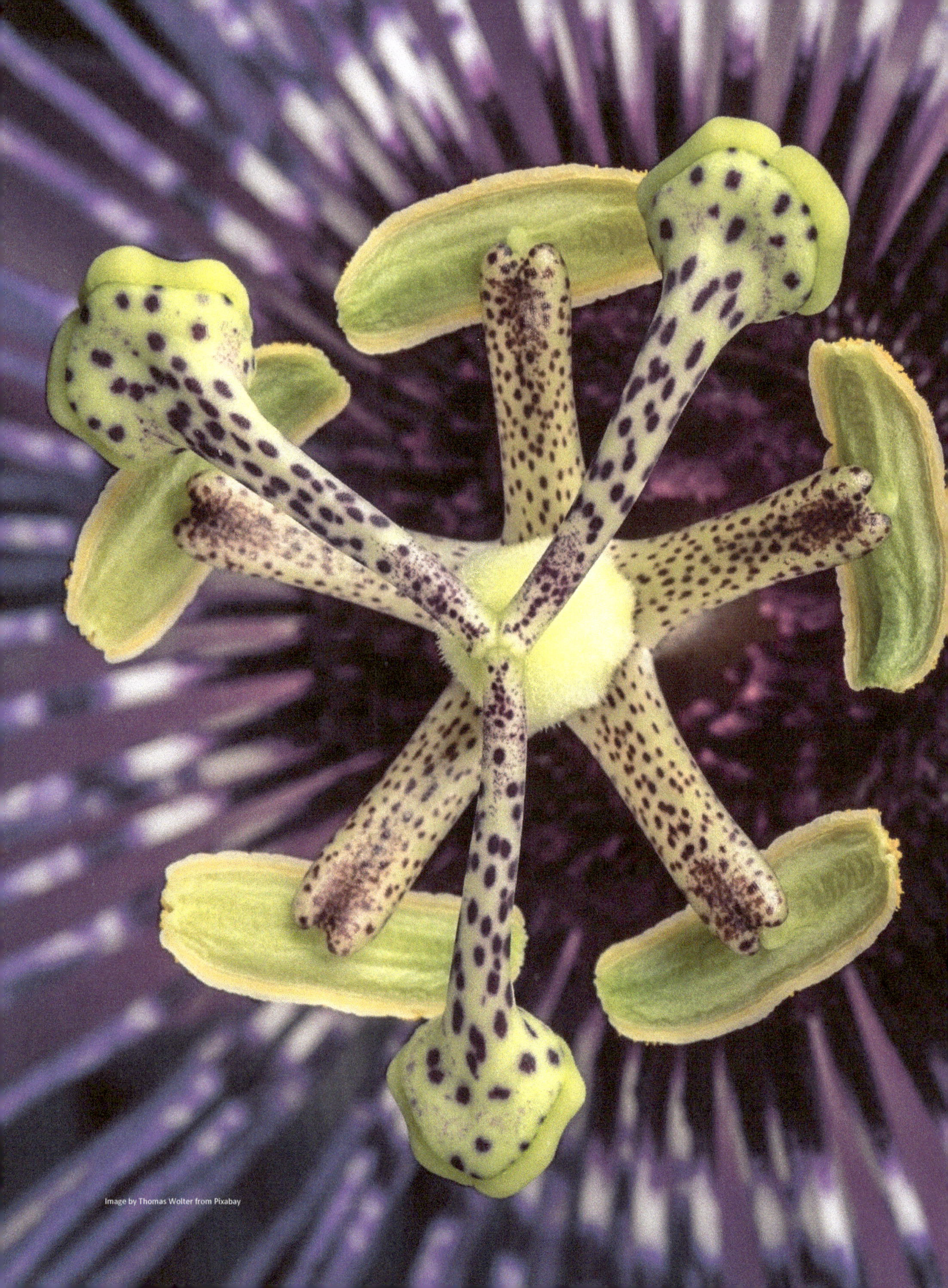

Image by Thomas Wolter from Pixabay

Passion fruit - Passiflora incarnata

Originating in Central and South America Passiflora incarnata is a member of a family with over 550 species and is now grown all over the world. Its members, known as Passiflora, have been found in Asia, Africa and Oceania and is the main herb used in the treatment of depression, anxiety and sleep disorders. It should be noted that some members of this family are also used in herbal medicine, but they contain detectable levels of cyanide and therefore any use should be discontinued. Passiflora foetida is one such species that has been shown to be toxic.

It is believed that the herb and fruit were introduced into Europe in the 17th century. Its flower has been given religious importance by Spanish Friars who brought it back from the Americas as they regarded it as a representation of the crucifixion. Today it is a well-known medicinal herb and is included in the database of the European Medicines Agency.

It is believed that the main chemical compounds responsible for the herbs anti-anxiety, anti-depressive and soporific attributes are harmaline, harman and harmalol. However, the precise understanding of how the herb works is still being researched.

In a study from Germany (2014) a group of 156 adults were given a dose of 425 mg of dried extract over 12 weeks. The researchers found a statistically significant reduction in anxiety, nervous restlessness and stress levels. They also measured the perceived Quality of Life response from the participants and found a considerable improvement.

Another research team, this time from Iran, compared the effects of the flower extract to the standard drugs imipramine and fluoxetine. Within this study, it was shown that the extract did indeed lessen depression. Another paper from 2016 also from Iran, sought to assess the effects of Passiflora incarnata extract in the treatment of General Anxiety Disorder (GAD). In this study, 30 patients aged between 18 and 24 were evaluated after 4 weeks. It was found that there was a statistically relevant improvement in the participants over this time. While this study was relatively small, it does go to increase the enormous body of work already carried out.

Research has also shown that the herb also reduces neuropathic pain sensation. As a result, it is useful in managing neuralgia and other chronic conditions.

Also, if you are having trouble in either getting to sleep or staying asleep, then Passiflora incarnata flower extract has been shown in a number of studies to improve the quality of sleep.

Putting it all together, it is clear that the wide-spread use of the flower extract from Passionfruit is supported and significant.

[1] H. Khan and S. M. Nabavi, "Passiflora (Passiflora incarnata)," Nonvitamin Nonmineral Nutr. Suppl., pp. 361–366, 2018.

[2] S. A. Maleki, "Evaluation of antidepressant-like effect of hydroalcoholic extract of Passiflora incarnata in animal models of depression in male mice," J. HerbMed Pharmacol. J. homepage J HerbMed Pharmacol, vol. 3, no. 1, pp. 41–45, 2014.

[3] J. Gibbert, F. Kreimendahl, J. Lebert, R. Rychlik, and I. Trompetter, "Improvement of Stress Resistance and Quality of Life of Adults with Nervous Restlessness after Treatment with a Passion Flower Dry Extract," Complement. Med. Res., vol. 24, no. 2, pp. 83–89, 2017.

[4] M. Nojoumi, P. Ghaeli, S. Salimi, A. Sharifi, and F. Raisi, "Effects of passion flower extract, as an add-on treatment to sertraline, on reaction time in patients with generalized anxiety disorder: A double-blind Placebo-controlled study," Iran. J. Psychiatry, vol. 11, no. 3, pp. 191–197, 2016.

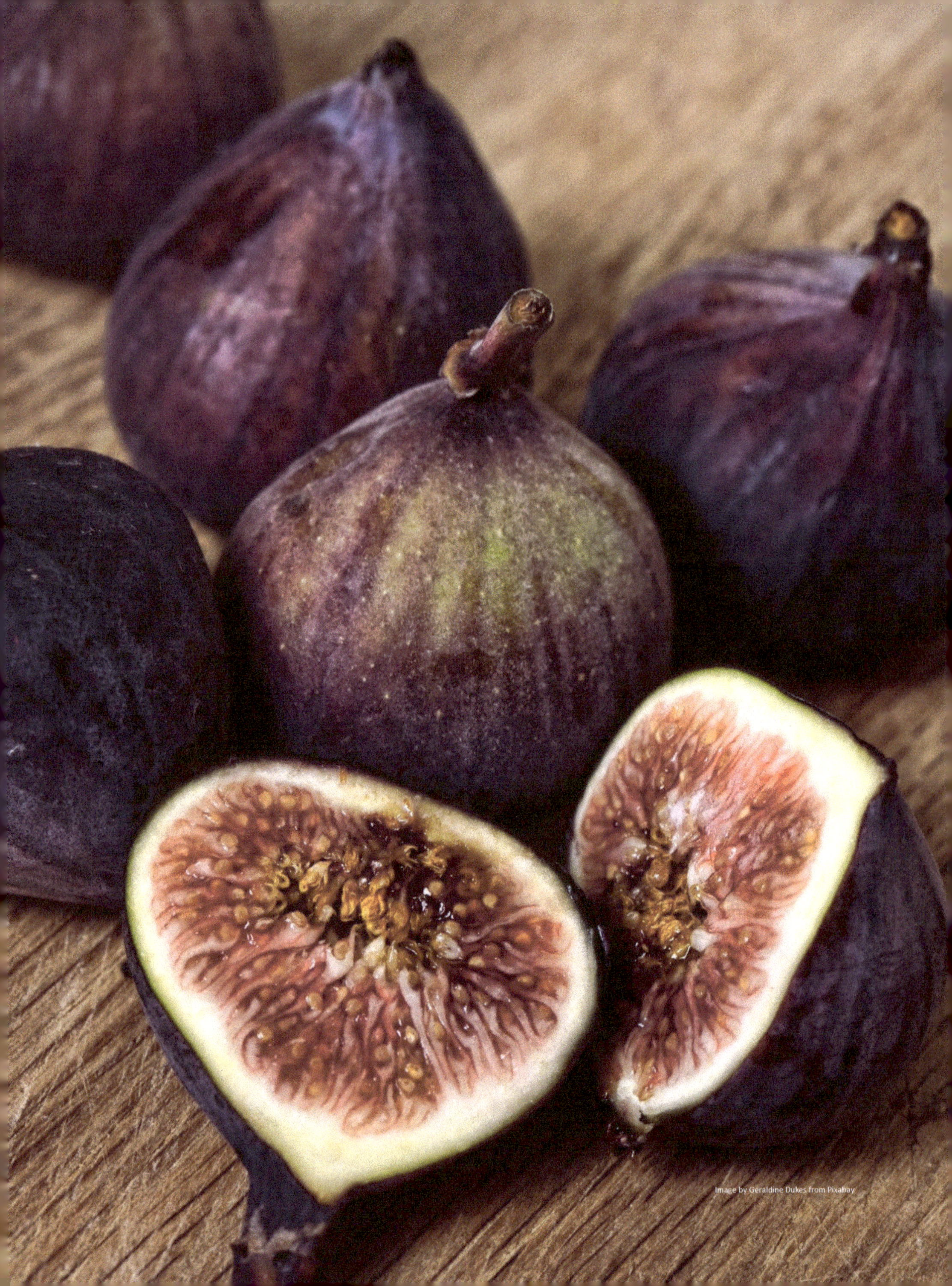

Image by Geraldine Dukes from Pixabay

Figs - Ficus religiosa

If there was one single tree that had to be in this book, then this is it! Worshipped for centuries in India and South East Asia the Ficus religiosa tree has a lot to be proud of. From being central to Hinduism and Jainism, the tree is also partially responsible for the commencement of Buddhism, so the stories about Siddhartha Gautama tell.

So, let's start at the beginning. Siddhartha Gautama was born a Prince, into a wealthy family in the Nepalese foothills of India. At his birth, the oracles and soothsayers all came to visit the new-born baby and predicted he would either become a famous King or holy man. Naturally, Siddhartha's father preferred the King option and as a result, kept the young prince locked up in his own palace and surrounded him with luxury and the satisfaction of any desire. At a young age Siddhartha was married to a beautiful young wife who bore him a son. However, not long after this, as the story goes, Siddhartha snuck out of the palace as he was utterly depressed and wanted to reconcile the world against the unfairness of it all. Once he was outside the palace, he saw that death came for all people, and for those in abject poverty it may have been a blessing, yet for both the rich and poor, it came all too quickly. So, he left to become a wandering Sadhu (penniless monk) to try and make sense of it all.

After many years he was becoming frustrated with his ascetic life and decided to sit in one spot until he had damned well figured it all out. As it so happened, he sat underneath a Ficus religiosa tree. By this stage, he had become mildly successful at being a penniless monk and had accumulated a few followers, but even they thought he had gone mad. So, they left him sitting there under the tree and he went begging for some better opportunities. As it happened on the morning of the 49th day, Siddhartha finally figured it all out and walked from the shade of the fig tree as an enlightened being or as he is better known, the Buddha. He was reported to be 35 years old at the time. The story continues that immediately after Siddhartha had gained Nirvana, he did not intend to teach it to anyone as he thought people were too full of ignorance, greed, and hatred. So not much has changed apparently! Anyway, he was convinced that he should teach his wisdom through Brahma Sahampati, and this is how we came to have Buddhism today.

Multiple research papers, all parts of the Fig tree have shown to be calmative, anti-anxiety and antidepressant. Extracts made from the bark, leaves and fruit of the tree have been reputed to be remedies for all manner of ailments, yet we are focused on the antidepressant aspect. Research from 2017 asserted that the fruit extract exhibited positive actions on the serotonin pathways. At doses of 300 mg/kilo of body weight, the effects were comparable to the standard antidepressants known as imipramine and fluoxetine. Other research from 2013 also sought to understand how the fruit extract reduced anxiety and depression, resulting in the same assumption that the extract influenced the serotonergic neurotransmission in the body. Incorporating common figs into diet can be expected to have a positive effect on depression as long as a minimum amount of 30 grams per serve is taken.

[1] B. Uma, K. Prabhakar, and S. Rajendran, "Invitro Antimicrobial Activity and Phytochemical Analysis of Ficus religiosa L . and Ficus bengalensis L . against Diarrhoeal Enterotoxigenic E . coli," Ethnobot. Leafl., vol. 13, no. 1, pp. 472–474, 2009.

[2] D. Paliwal, K. Murti, Y. Sangwan, M. Kaushik, and D. Kiran, "ewsletter Paliwal et al . PRELIMI ARY A D PHARMACOLOGICAL PROFILE OF FICUS RELIGIOSA L .: A OVERVIEW Paliwal et al .," Pharmacologyonline, vol. 395, pp. 387–395, 2011.

[3] A. Kaur, A. C. Rana, V. Tiwari, R. Sharma, and S. Kumar, "Review on ethanomedicinal and pharmacological properties of Ficus religiosa," J. Appl. Pharm. Sci., vol. 1, no. 8, pp. 6–11, 2011.

[4] S. A. Bhalerao and A. S. Sharma, "Original Research Article Ethenomedicinal , phytochemical and pharmacological profile of Ficus religiosa Roxb," vol. 3, no. 11, pp. 528–538, 2014.

[5] R. Rutuja, U. Shivsharan, and A. Shruti, "Ficus Religiosa (Peepal): A Phytochemical and Pharmacological Review," Int. J. Pharm. Chem. Sci., vol. 4, no. 3, pp. 360–370, 2015.

[6] E. B. Devanesan, A. Vijaya Anand, P. S. Kumar, P. Vinayagamoorthy, and P. Basavaraju, "Phytochemistry and Pharmacology of Ficus religiosa," Syst. Rev. Pharm., vol. 9, no. 1, pp. 45–48, 2018.

[7] J. O. Bhangale and S. R. Acharya, "Anti-Parkinson Activity of Petroleum Ether Extract of Ficus religiosa (L .) Leaves," vol. 2016, 2016.

Introduction

"Once you're grown up you can't come back"

Peter Pan

There are various things to know about depression, and then forget them. They are all just far too depressing. The therapy, the counselling, the medications, and the friends who think they know what you are experiencing. This is not to say that these things are bad. It's just that they do not seem to work, most of the time. However, there is good news and as they say bad news. So, let's deal with the bad news first ...... You, or someone you know is depressed. Now that that is out of the way, onto the good news ...... You, or your friend, is most probably artistic, witty, caring and definitely not a psychopath, sociopath, nor stupid.

It is estimated that during this decade depression will be the single largest cause of disability on the planet. A report from the World Health Organisation estimates that there are over 300 million cases of people suffering from depression. When we consider that these are recognized cases, then with unreported incidents it may be far higher. Another disturbing estimate is that the rate of suicide in adolescents and young adults (15-29 years of age) is 30 times higher if they suffer from depression. This in itself is an extraordinary statement, as wouldn't you have to be somewhat unhappy in order to kill yourself? To my knowledge, no one ever in history has decided to end it all because they were deliriously happy.

The reality of depression is that it changes you. It makes you see things you wish you hadn't, and then you wonder why no one else sees them. But, now that you have experienced another world view, you are not like other people, and most likely will never be again. Just like the red pill and the blue pill in the movie Matrix, once you choose one, you can never go back. You simply learn to cope with the change, and if you are good at it, make it work for you.

The other good news is that in order to be depressed, you probably have a higher IQ than most people. So, you're smart. At this point a depressed person will most likely dismiss this as irrelevant by saying, "Well if I am so damned smart, then why can't I stop being depressed!?"

Which is to say, "You're stupid and leave me alone. Can't you see I am depressed!" Herein lies the paradox of depression; to be depressed you have to be really, really smart, as this is the only way you can argue against every possible conversation you have with yourself on why you should not be depressed, and win. Ergo sum, you are smart. If you were stupid, you would simply say "I can't be depressed because I like butterflies, fishing, home-made cookies and online shopping". Which is to say easily distracted. Depressive people are tenacious. They are determined, and they are successful in being miserable, despite everything. They simply can't stop thinking and ensuring that they are less than everything else.

So, that positive can be claimed, yet ironically our intelligence is also our jailor to a certain extent. Imagine if you can, two adversaries that are equally matched in every way in strength, intelligence, endurance and even appearance. Who will win? Will their contest end? Will it matter? Now imagine that there are two of you.
This is precisely the issue we are facing. Depressives battle their own logic! Or to put it more clearly, we try and outsmart ourselves, which is an almost impossible situation with which to create a positive outcome from, and which more often than not results in stagnation, and ergo sum: depression. The more intelligent you are, the more convincing and complex the internal debate is of why you should not be, and why you should be ... happy.

What exactly is depression?

In one way, it is an intellectual space. An area where only you can be and everyone else is outside. You know that you are deserving of love, deserving of success, and worthy of happiness. It's just that you know precisely how to stop yourselves from achieving it, and unable to stop yourselves from destroying it. Depression is unique to each person, and therefore a depressive person will not try and convince fellow depressive that they know what they are going through ... 'cause they don't! Depression is like a fingerprint, and unique to the individual. All we can do is say, 'Yeah, I know what you mean', and then hang with our depressed friend and talk about other stuff.

It's that simple companionship. The acknowledgement of 'I am not alone in my dungeon anymore' is often the most effective support for the sufferer in achieving a balance in life. We can share experiences, but we cannot pretend we know what the other is feeling, other than it being some form of emptiness and self-decay. We can hang together whilst we watch the world move on and not give a shit about us. Which of course it shouldn't, but we resent it anyway.

Depression is full of irony, satire, and liberal sprinkles of oxymorons. Never in the history of medicine have so many people, from all races, cultures, and socio-economic layers considered themselves to be alone or isolated. With a combined population mass rapidly approaching a snug 8 billion, the percentage of people suffering from depression and anxiety is increasing. So, why, with our ever-increasing numbers, do more and more of us feel alone?

The facts are hard to pin down. One report confidently states that approximately 21% of the global population suffers from depression. Such a bold statement was not in some tabloid, nor internet blog, but found in a scientific research paper on depression from 2008. In another research paper it was claimed that 20% of the population of the USA suffers from some form of depressive symptomology. So, let's just stop here. Going any further would have a more disparate and confusing numbers thrown at us. Let's just accept that there are a lot of us who are ... how would we say ... a little bit blue.

21% of the global population is a big number and if this is correct then 1.5 billion people are currently sad and depressed. That is roughly 1 in 5 people. So theoretically if you find yourself depressed at a party where there are 50 odd people, chances are 10 of you would have something in common.

Depression has invisible velvet handcuffs that we help fit to size, and then remain unable to free ourselves from even when the lock is obviously broken. Depression is the ability to stare out of the window of the future with all its possibilities and say, "Well, that's boring!"

Depression is also powerful and full of beauty. I should know I have been depressed for forty years and have become quite an expert in having conversations with my adversary.

Ultimately, depression is not fun, and it is more real in some ways than nearly everything else. It is a paradox of the desperate desire to change, in bed with the futility of eternity.

Isolation is the hallmark of depression. We don't want it. We know what we are doing. If there is a hell, then depressed people are not afraid of it, as anything must be better than where we are. At least hell has group activities and demons to blame.

So, if it's all doom and gloom, then why bother with a book?

My answer is three-fold. Over time I have become convinced that depression is not correctly or fairly dealt with. We are labelling depressive people as if they are defective, but in truth, depressives are some of the most influential and optimistic people on the planet. Think of Abraham Lincoln, Carl Jung, Vincent van Gogh, and Dwayne the Rock Johnson.

One even started a religion. However, the followers demand it merely is a philosophy. They do this because they are a bit dark in their point of view. However, any system that makes you wake up at 5 am to pray is no longer a philosophy but a structured system for abasement and control. But I digress, let's continue.

Secondly, I like to share my long-standing interest in scientific research into herbal medicines, and especially for depression and anxiety. They have a gentle impact, few side effects, are low cost, and less intrusive to the body than the pharmaceutical medications prescribed. As a young man I studied under Dorothy Hall, one of Australia's leading and most experienced herbalists.

Thirdly, my own experience with depression and what I have learned can possibly assist others.

I remember many decades ago when I was a young man struggling with life, I had the wonderful luck to meet a friend who I found over time had one of the best minds and highest IQs I had ever met. Even now, James is still one of my dearest friends and retains his prodigious intellect. However, way back then, a century ago, we met and saw within each of us a kindred spirit in the world of depression. Long, smoke and wine-filled evenings discussing the meaning of life ensued with no solution emerging as to how or why depression penetrates the soul. One day, James related to me a story of a person he met at some social gathering or other. The person intrigued James in the same way as if an alien had quietly walked into a wedding reception and calmly asked for a glass of wine. James put it this way. "As I was bouncing quietly around the crowd, I came upon this man, and we struck up one of those polite stranger conversations. He said he worked in a factory down near Botany within the southern suburbs of Sydney. On the weekends he told me he liked to go fishing. He told me about his wife and children, one of whom suffers from a low-grade chronic illness, of which I have forgotten the name. Anyway, as he talked there seemed to be something extraordinary about this guy. I thought I would ask him if he ever thought about the meaning of life. You know, just testing how deep the water was. He just stared at me. So, I asked again, and he then asked me as to what did I mean? I said again "You know.... life, the universe, and everything. Don't you wonder what it all means?" He thought for a second and replied, "No, I never really thought about it!". Now it was my turn to stare. Here was a man that enjoyed his job, loved his wife and children. He had simple hobbies and didn't appear to be overly ambitious. He just seemed really really, happy!" After James had stopped telling me of the encounter, we were quiet for a while. A happy man! Who would have thought that such a creature actually existed? I then asked James, "Since meeting this guy, have you ever thought you would like to be like him?" James turned to me in horror and laughed out "Of course not!" "Why?", I pursued. "Well," replied James, "For a start, he was a fucking moron!"

It was around this time that I answered a question that I did not know I had. If, to get over my depression, I had to truly become a simple and basic person, would I do it? I found myself agreeing with James, no, not on my life! So, in some roundabout way, I realised that I myself had chosen depression, and in this simple realization I became a damned site more powerful than having depression inflicted on me. Ever since, if the alternative to depression was being a stupid moron, then this was not attractive and so my adventure into dungeons, labyrinths and dark forests began. As I dove into depression, I surprisingly found positives are hiding within it, in our inner prisons. The association between intelligence and depression is one such that James made clear to me. One of many papers published in 2017 in Scientific American undeniably concluded that smarter people have a higher probability of entering or suffering depression. From Aristotle to Einstein, history is peppered with examples of men and women gifted with genius and cursed with melancholy. As Bertrand Russell so eloquently stated, "The whole problem with the world is that fools and fanatics are so sure of themselves, and wiser people are so full of doubts!".

The Little Termites was a term used to describe a group of highly gifted children with IQ's over 170 that were studied over many years starting in the 1960s and into the 1990s. One of the outcomes from the study was a clear link between intelligence and a lack of satisfaction in life. It was also found that intelligent people worried excessively, but not merely about their own life trajectory, they also worried about the world at large and were annoyed by egotistical, irrational, and illogical behaviour. If you also worry in such a way, then there is chance that you have a well above average IQ.

One paradox we must deal with is the question why people, less intelligent than us, hold positions superior to us? There may be two explanations as to why your boss is excruciatingly stupid or despotic. One is called the Dunning-Kruger effect and defines at which point someone is so stupid that they cannot self-evaluate themselves. In this paradigm, to assess your own skills or abilities you require precisely the same level of intelligence to be able to carry out these skills. A competent person good at their work is therefore able to review their actions and thus their performance. In the Dunning-Kruger argument, the stupid person cannot possibly understand how bad they are at something as they lack the necessary intelligence required to do a good job. This results in stupid people thinking that they are actually brilliant at their tasks resulting in them believing that they deserve advancement in a field or career.

The other reason is that they are either a psychopath or sociopath. Both terms are mostly interchangeable. So, as you are depressed and constantly self-evaluate, you are neither stupid nor a psychopath, yet you are also retarding your advancement when compared to these others because you think you don't deserve the elevation or suffer internal criticism where you think you might not be able to. This is why at the top of corporations and governments we find both the Dunning-Kruger effect and the behaviour of charming madmen and women.

The realization that you need to develop other skills to imbalance the internal debate becomes more evident. Further, in acute cases of depression, the use of medicines, either herbal or pharmaceutical become necessary. Our demons, as we find out, are very intelligent little devils precisely because we have made them that way. Therefore, we need other weapons by which to contain them. Currently, today, there are numerous methods or therapies with which to combat depression.

One of these methods is called art therapy and it has been used for several decades as an attempt to either alleviate depression or understand it or both. The premise arose out of the perceived link between famous artists and their own sorrows. Think Vincent van Gogh, or Edvard Munch, or Jackson Pollack, all of whom suffered from acute depression. Researchers sought to understand whether to make genuinely great art, you had to be depressed first. This is called the creativity-mood disorder based on the assumption that mood, primarily negative moods such as bi-polar disorder, are necessary for the creation of art. In this context, art encompasses all aspects of music, graphic design, painting etc. An article from 2018 published in the magazine of the British Psychological Society discussed the findings from a recent meta-analysis of prior research into this question. As it was, the results were contradictory, with some studies showing a clear association of creativity accompanying mood disorders such as bi-polar, and another group of data having a less clear outcome. The article posed the hypothesis that to create art, the artists are required to be able to review their work and draw upon past experiences and emotions. Here again, the Dunning-Kruger effect comes into play as this would be impossible for a stupid person.

So, our wandering across this ocean of ennui reveals that a depressed person has a much higher chance of being both intelligent and creative. This means that with intent we can draw upon our creative side, use it as a tool to release our frustrations, dark thoughts, and conflicting emotions, thereby reducing the impact of our depression!

Many causes of depression have been recognized, or perhaps a better term would be 'triggers of depression', and they include post-traumatic stress disorder (PTSD), sexual abuse, assault, broken families, abusive parents, school bullying, disease, and even the unknown slow infection into the otherwise everyday life of emptiness and loneliness. Whatever the trigger, if/when the event actually passes, and you are clearly alive still (which in itself is cause for optimism) than sadly enough surviving the trigger event more often than not was not the end of the torture. For instance, a sexual assault ten years ago can, and often does, still manifest in the survivor's mind as either fear or depression, or both. The book is about the emotion of depression, and how to manage depression to a point where depression is no longer your master. Instead, you will master your depression through understanding the influences surrounding you and connecting with positive aspects of life with the use of herbs. This book is all about breaking depression down into 'the bad is not so bad', and that 'the good is, well .. liveable'.

Actually, in every traditional culture, there have been herbs to remedy depression. Thus, we must realize that depression is not a modern condition, but that it has afflicted men and women for thousands of years. Over time, through trial and error or just dumb luck, a library of effective botanic cures or aids has been created. The most effective herbs are provided within this book.

Science has found physical anomalies in the brain and also in the hormone levels of depressed people which have resulted in the development of many of our antidepressant drugs that we utilize seeking to address these chemical and physiological imbalances with varying degrees of success. The big question here is whether the physical manifestations of the depressive state are the causes or the symptoms of it. As an example, let's imagine an average relatively happy person who suffers from a sudden horrific event that spans several weeks. The death of a loved one perhaps. After some time, they are diagnosed with depression due to the event. It is clear that the person did not suffer from any physical trauma, only emotional and psychological. So, any physical changes to their endocrine system or neuronal integrity were caused by the emotional event. By treating this person's body with antidepressant drugs is clearly the treatment of symptoms, not the cause. Obviously, such a person would also have to engage in psychological or psychiatric therapy in order to resolve the emotional pain of losing their loved one in an intellectual manner. Drugs would not be able to cure alone.

It would be fair to state that depression and anxiety are two defining health conditions of our time. In truth, we actually know very little of the causes, and therefore our treatments are not as effective and/or dangerous. As Abraham Maslow coined in his book *The Psychology of Science*, "When all one has is a hammer, everything looks like a nail!"

By the way, this book is not intended to replace the current medication you might already be on. This book rather is to give the depressed, or those not already under treatment for depression, or those living with a depressed more tools by which to cope. The plants listed within these pages have all been rigorously studied and may offer anyone a more holistic solution with far fewer side effects. Yet, they are not intended to be a replacement for therapy advised by a medical practitioner, but rather more a complementary suite of herbal medicines.

Furthermore, every chapter in these pages end with references so you may get enticed to further reading.

Lastly, long have various animal totems been associated with emotions or skill sets. We can be as wise as an owl, or have a memory like an elephant, or are referred to with 'don't worry about Fred he is just a big lovable bear'. For depression, we ended up with a dog. More specifically, a black dog, and some people have gone further and claim the dog is a Labrador. The origin of the depressive mascot is thought to have come from Sir Winston Churchill who often stated that he was "walking the black dog", his metaphor for the times when he was suffering bouts of dark and gloomy mood. It is now almost universally associated with the condition.

So, how can we get the black dog to do what we want?

We get inside the dog - to see, feel, hear, smell, walk it to train it.

[1] Q. Liu, H. He, J. Yang, X. Feng, F. Zhao, and J. Lyu, "Changes in the global burden of depression from 1990 to 2017: Findings from the Global Burden of Disease study," J. Psychiatr. Res., vol. 126, no. August 2019, pp. 134–140, 2019.

[2] N. Tagalidou, E. Distlberger, V. Loderer, and A. R. Laireiter, "Efficacy and feasibility of a humor training for people suffering from depression, anxiety, and adjustment disorder: A randomized controlled trial," BMC Psychiatry, vol. 19, no. 1, pp. 1–13, 2019.

[3] U. Willinger et al., "Cognitive and emotional demands of black humour processing: the role of intelligence, aggressiveness and mood," Cogn. Process., vol. 18, no. 2, pp. 159–167, 2017.

[4] 北村純一 et al., "1. 顔面麻痺タイプの診断に難渋した1症例 (第1回 日本リハビリテーション医学会関東地方会)," Japanese J. Rehabil. Med., vol. 34, no. 3, pp. 234–235, 1997.

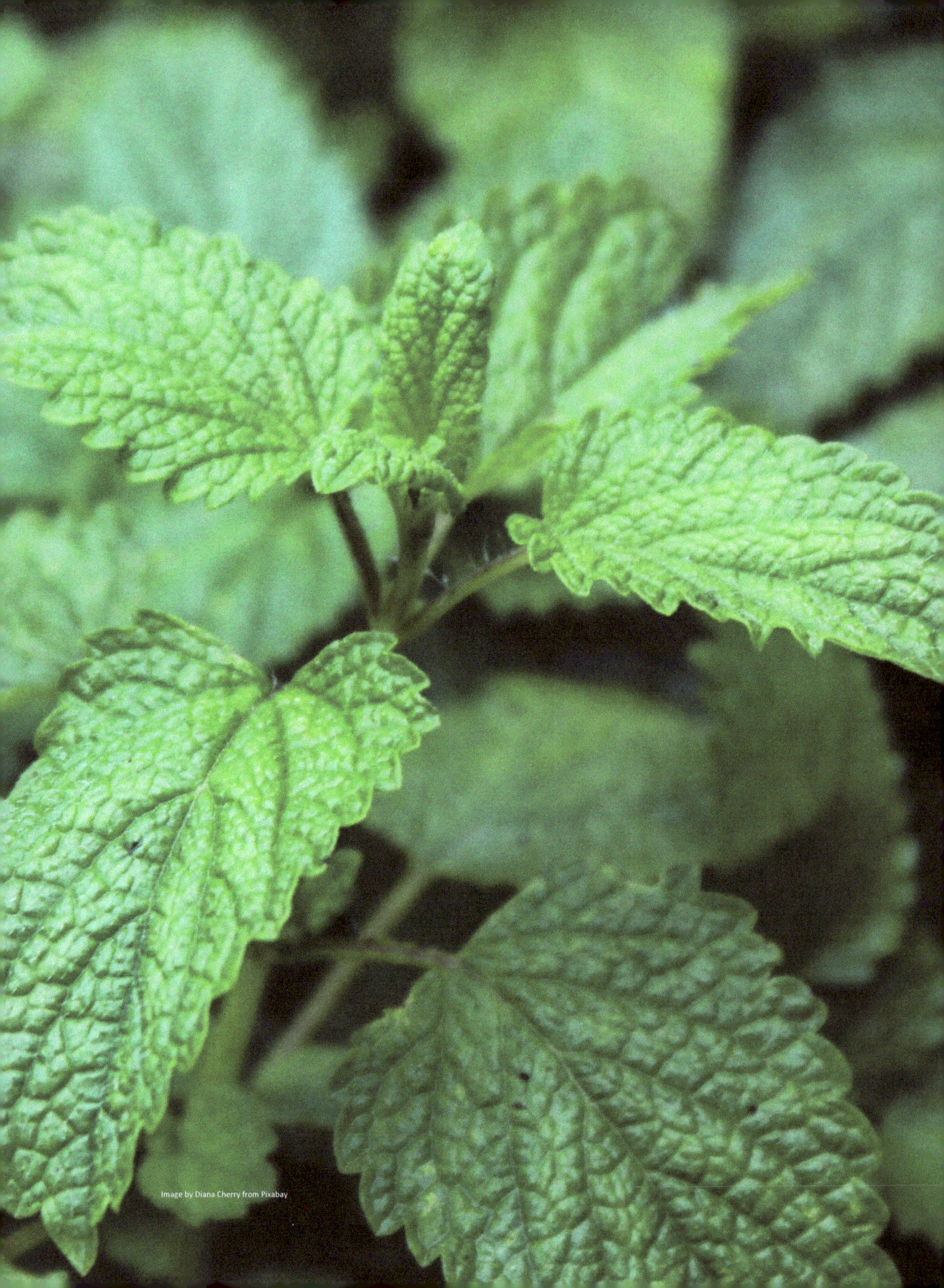

Image by Diana Cherry from Pixabay

Lemon Balm - Melissa officinalis

In the first century, one of the most outstanding physicians of the Islamic Golden age was a proponent of the use of Lemon Balm. Ibn Sina, also known as Avicenna, was a prolific polymath and his famous manuscript on medicine known as the Canon of Medicine was used throughout the Islamic and European medieval world up until the 17th century. (actor Ben Kingsley plays Sina in 2013 movie The Physician) Paracelsus, one of Europe's leading physicians in the early 16th century probably had a copy and he called Lemon Balm the Elixir of Life. Its scientific name is Melissa originates from the Greek meaning honeybee, it is also the name of the Greek nymph who discovered honey and who nursed the infant Zeus according to mythology. Therefore, with such a long and acclaimed history Lemon Balm should be all it is reported to be.

Traditionally used as an antibacterial, antiviral, gastrointestinal tonic, anti-anxiety, antidepressant, an improver of cognitive function and sleep patterns. Recent research has supported Lemon Balm in the management of Alzheimer's disease.

A research paper from 2009 compared the aqueous (water) extract from its leaves as well as the essential oil of the plant to the standard antidepressant drugs imipramine and fluoxetine. In this paper, the researchers found a significant improvement in depression when compared to these drugs. Administration of the oil via an injection into the peritoneal cavity (abdominal cavity) had the most significant improvement in the test animals, indicating that taking the oil orally would be equally as effective.

Another paper (2012) compared the ethanol extract from the leaves of Lemon Balm for anxiety as well as depression and found it to be effective in reducing both. This study used diazepam as well as fluoxetine as standard drug comparatives. It was found that a dose of 300 mg/kg body weight was the optimal dose. Interestingly, this paper discussed the differences in gender, where females reacted more positively to Lemon Balm than the males, indicating the rarely discussed aspects of different aetiology (characteristics) for men and women suffering from depression and anxiety.

A more recent study (2018) aimed to compare Lemon Balm against chamomile in the treatment of depression. It found that both were effective in reducing the symptoms of depression. Therefore, combining the two herbs will have a greater result than using them as a single treatment.

Discussions surrounding the use of Lemon Balm also indicate its effectiveness in promoting energy and activity. As a result, the plant may be thought of as an adaptogen or general tonic. The daily use of the leaves of the plant in a simple tisane (tea) may be recommended for any person undergoing stressful conditions.

Many research papers have supported the use of Lemon Balm to increase brain function or cognition in both learning and memory.

[1] M. Emamghoreishi and M. S. Talebianpour, "Antidepressant effect of melissa officinalis in the forced swimming test," Daru, vol. 17, no. 1, pp. 42–47, 2009.

[2] B. S, "Phyto-Pharmacological Effect of Nine Medicinal Plants as a Traditional Treatment on Depression," J. Appl. Pharm., vol. 09, no. 03, 2017.

[3] A. Shakeri, A. Sahebkar, and B. Javadi, "Melissa officinalis L. - A review of its traditional uses, phytochemistry and pharmacology," J. Ethnopharmacol., vol. 188, pp. 204–228, 2016.

[4] E. A. Moacă et al., "A Comparative Study of Melissa officinalis Leaves and Stems Ethanolic Extracts in terms of Antioxidant, Cytotoxic, and Antiproliferative Potential," Evidence-based Complement. Altern. Med., vol. 2018, pp. 11–14, 2018.

[5] A. Namjou, N. Yazdani, E. Abbasi, and M. Rafieian-Kopaei, "The antidepressant activity of matricaria chamomilla and melissa officinalis ethanolic extracts in non-reserpinized and reserpinized Balb/C Mice," Jundishapur J. Nat. Pharm. Prod., vol. 13, no. 4, 2018.

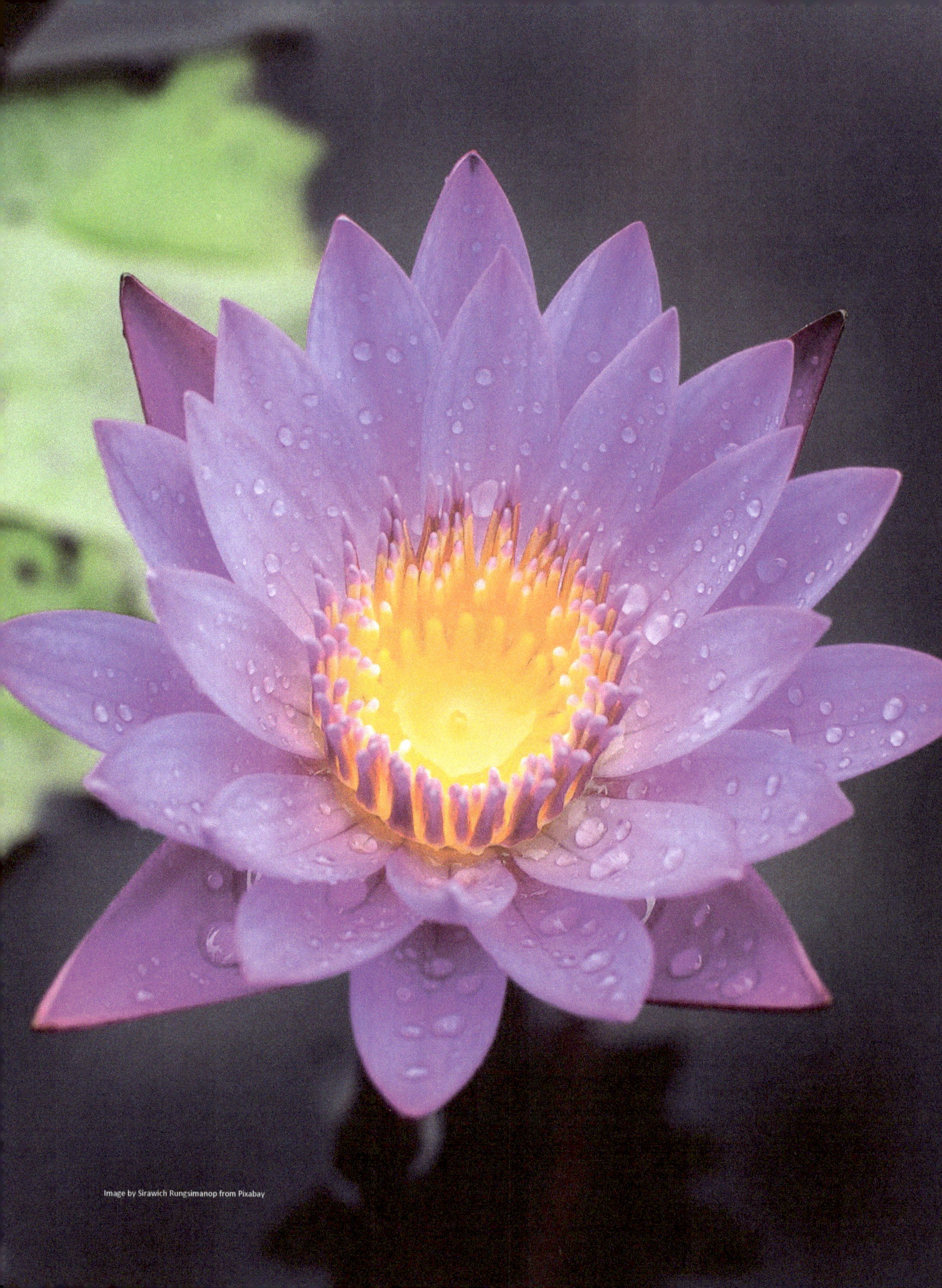

Image by Sirawich Rungsimanop from Pixabay

Water Lily / Lotus - Nymphaea lotus

All Water Lilies and Lotuses fall into the Nymphaeaceae family, except for the Holy Lotus Nelumbo nucifera which has been removed and placed in its own unique family. Yet all the lilies and lotuses, including Nelumbo nucifera, share similar medicinal actions and uses. One quick way of telling the Nymphaeaceae apart from its Nelumbo cousins is that the Holy Lotus has a perfectly circular leaf and others have a cleft penetrating to the central stem of the leaf. Also, the apparent distinction between what is a Lily and Lotus is that the Lotus flower is held several centimetres above the surface of the water whilst the Lily flower floats on the surface.

The Water Lily and Lotus have been cultivated as food and medicine for thousands of years. In many cultures the plant is used in rituals and ceremonies due to the mild psychoactive effects it has once eaten or drunk as a tea. Throughout the regions where they are found they have been harvested as food as the leaves are used as a green vegetable, and roots as a starch. China is the largest producer of Lotus root, yet this is almost purely N. nucifera.

Lilies and Lotuses contain apomorphine and nuciferine. Apomorphine has been described as a psychoactive alkaloid and is a non-selective dopamine agonist. It is primarily used to treat Parkinson's disease as it stimulates dopamine receptors and improves motor function. Nuciferine is an alkaloid associated with dopamine receptor blockade. A 2013 paper on the antidepressant actions of the Nymphaea alba flower showed that doses of 200 mg/kg body weight were more effective than imipramine in reducing depression like symptoms in laboratory animals. The Blue Lotus, Nymphaea caerulea, is one of the most widely used members of this family due to its use as a mild psychoactive stimulant. It can be found in many alternative health food outlets where it is sold as a tisane (tea) and more recently as a vape. In certain nations, the use of this plant is 'controlled', and it would be wise to find out the laws in your area before using it.

The apomorphine compound is pharmaceutically mass-produced and used in various situations. Currently, it is recommended in the management of Parkinson's disease and also for drug addiction. In veterinary practices it is used as an emetic for dogs suspected of poisoning. The compound, even though it sounds similar to morphine, has no morphine structures in it and does not act like an opioid.

Other research from 2016 also confirmed that the plant is an effective anti-anxiety and depression medication. In this research from a combined effort from universities in America, Brazil and Nigeria showed that the simple aqueous leaf extract from Nymphaea lotus was effective, however not as effective as the standard drug used as a control during the experiments, which has diazepam.

Pregnant women should not use Nymphaea extracts as they act as uterotonics inducing contraction and may act as abortifacients.

[1] J. L. Poklis et al., "HHS Public Access," vol. 49, no. 3, pp. 175–181, 2018.

[2] J. O. Fajemiroye, K. Adam, K. Zjawiony Jordan, C. E. Alves, and A. A. Aderoju, "Evaluation of anxiolytic and antidepressant-like activity of aqueous leaf extract of nymphaea lotus linn. In mice," Iran. J. Pharm. Res., vol. 17, no. 2, pp. 613–626, 2018.

[3] a R. On, S. Of, and H. Formulation, "International Journal of Phytotherapy," Int. J. Phyther., vol. 2, no. 2, pp. 74–88, 2012.

[4] A. A. Of and E. Extract, "Anti-Depressant Activity of Ethanolic Extract of," vol. 4, no. 5. pp. 382–385, 2013.

[5] N. Africa, T. Asia, and L. Concern, "Nymphaea alba - Nilofar," pp. 3–5.

The science so far

"I was depressed at that time. I was in analysis. I was suicidal as a matter of fact and would have killed myself, but I was in analysis with a strict Freudian, and, if you kill yourself, they make you pay for the sessions you miss"

Woody Allen

In this chapter, we will strive to understand where the science sits concerning the analysis of depression. Yet, I can tell you right now the science is quite messy. In fact, it is quite depressing, excuse the pun. When I started research into herbs and their effectiveness in treating or ameliorating depression, I found that the scientific research did not provide enough understanding of this complex condition. I sought a wider narrative on how the herbs can assist with all aspects of its causes to understand and alleviate depression. All aspects had to be analysed for the book to be worthwhile.

So, I started my dive into Dr Google. I started reading many papers on the aetiology of depression, the cause, set of causes, or manner of causation of a disease or condition. I can sum my research up with a report from 2015 that states that "the causes of depression are fuzzy and heterogeneous". The term heterogeneous basically means 'of random causes or diverse influences.' And it appeared that many articles on the topic of depression have a similar disclaimer. This made me realise that if this is the case, then our treatments of depression can also be random at best. And hence should it be any surprise that many people do not benefit from the current pharmaceutical regimes employed by both medical and psychiatric doctors?

Furthermore, this condition is rapidly becoming one of the most significant health challenges of our modern time!

I also learned that researchers and therapists are still debating what category to place depression in. Is depression a disease, a syndrome, a condition or a disorder? The most straight forward answer would be 'all of the above'. However, science wants to place a framework around this condition so that outcomes on symptomatology and treatment can be more precise. This was exactly the issue discussed in the paper from 2015 titled *"Problematic assumptions have slowed down depression research: why symptoms not syndromes are the way forward"*. Its authors argued that for diagnosis and treatments, it would be more effective if depression were thought of as a disease. Unfortunately, this was the paper that concluded that causes of depression are 'fuzzy' at best. Presently, it appears that the causes of depression are split into two factors.

One states it is genetic. It is believed that approximately 35+% of people suffer from depression because they have inherited the condition from their parents. The other factor attributes the cause to the environment or environmental factors such as diet, pollution, learnt behaviour, work, stress, sleep etc. A first reaction to the genetic imperfection theory is to surrender to the immutable influence, that it is something we cannot change. This is patently not true however. By believing it is purely in your genes is as much a cop out as saying 'I give up, I can't change it'. When we look at the genetic paradigm there are two aspects to consider. Firstly, and most importantly, this diagnosis has not been proven. A gene or a genetic sequence that is clearly a cause for depression has not been discovered yet. Therefore, the genetic causation is at best merely an assumption. Secondly, if depression is caused by genetic makeup, then we must consider it in conjunction with a multitude of other contributing factors that are genetic. You might be more susceptible to stress, you might be allergic to gluten and hence inflammatory reactions associated with it, or you might have smaller or larger regions in your brain compared to others. There are many different genetic compositions just as there are unique fingerprints. As an example, eye colour, which in and of itself, does not cause depression but might make you more prone to suffering from it as you have not compensated for your genetic variance as you simply do not know what this variance is. Some researchers argue in favour of the genetic causes of depression if you have had one or both of your parents suffer from depression. However, a child growing up in a home with a depressive parent is just as likely to 'learn' depressive tendencies. Furthermore, scientific research identified clear links to other influences for depression. They are:

- Diet
- Electromagnetic pollution
- Stress
- Inflammation
- Intelligence
- Trauma either physical, emotional or both
- Environmental pollution
- Illness
- Finance
- Age
- The information age (internet of things)
- And even gender (more women suffer from depression)

Simply tick off categories that you think apply to you in this list, and a rudimentary outline or plan will emerge. For example, a young girl of above-average intelligence, is gluten intolerant, spends a great deal of time on social media is diagnosed with suffering depression. The list of influences provides a clearer understanding of how the factors impact her depression. Some of these factors require no explanation, yet others do, such as diet and electro-pollution.

Naturally, a person who is on a regime of antidepressants may not receive the full benefit from drugs if diet or inflammatory conditions etc have not been addressed as well.

As we acquire a broader understanding of the possible causes of depression, we can become even more confused when discussing the various types of depression. We find depression is not a one size fits all, as science has identified many divergent types. There is even a type defined as Seasonal Adjusted Depression with the coined acronym SAD. I am not sure if the researcher who coined this term spent hours thinking of the best name so that the acronym could be formed, or they were not really serious about it. Imagine using it in conversation 'I'm depressed because I am or have SAD'. No, you are depressed because you hate long cold, dark winters!

A medical diagnosis defines the various depressive states as 'mild to severe' with unique characteristics. Let's string them all together in one paragraph. A person may start with Mild Depression (MD) which may persist for an extended time and become dysthymia or Persistent Depressive Disorder (PDD) accompanied by anhedonia or the lack of feeling pleasure. Should this continue, it may then be diagnosed as Major Depressive Disorder (MDD). Things may turn for the worse and the sufferer may then be thought of as having Psychotic Depression (PD). If you are a woman this entire process may be triggered by Post-Partum Depression (PPD), however, if you have not had a baby (as a man this is highly unlikely other than the case of Thomas Beatie the first transgender man to give birth), then this all may have been caused by a traumatic event thereby giving rise to Post Traumatic Stress Disorder (PTSD). However, if you are a woman and have not given birth, the trigger may have arisen from Premenstrual Dysphoric Disorder (PDD), yet if you suffered from Disruptive Mood Dysregulation Disorder (DMDD) as a child, then it may have started very early. After all of this, you may simply have Atypical Depression (AD), but it also may be Manic Depression (MD) or Bipolar Disorder (BD).

There are several other types that we can add to this list, however, this will only serve to confuse us even more. For the sake of simplicity, this book doesn't pick any favourites and will treat it all as simply depression.

Let's now add even more complexity with the research into the physical aspects of depression. It brings us to the age-old question concerning the chicken and the egg, and which one came first. Are the imbalances in the body the cause of depression, or does depression cause these imbalances in the body? On this question, the jury is still out. However, other than the genetic possible cause of depression, the bulk of the causes discussed earlier are all external influences, and the logic would therefore assume that these external impacts stimulate the imbalances in the body. The main physical imbalances that science and therapy focus on deal with the neurotransmitters or chemical agents that regulate how the body works. The main ones are serotonin, dopamine and norepinephrine, all of which are monoamines. These chemicals transmit messages across nerve cells. Serotonin is known as the happy chemical, dopamine is known as the pleasure chemical and norepinephrine is known as the flight or fight chemical. The monoamine theory of depression asserts that low levels of these neurotransmitters create depression, however, this theory is still considered controversial even though the majority of antidepressant pharmaceuticals target these chemical imbalances, and they are the main medications administered by therapists.

Mostly, depression is managed by prescribing a suite of antidepressants. They fit into a few basic categories being:

- Selective Serotonin Reuptake Inhibitors (SSRI), to delay or reduce the amount of serotonin reabsorbed by the body, and thereby increasing the levels of this monoamine.
- Dopamine and SNRI much the same as the SSRI except they also increase the levels of norepinephrine.
- Tricyclic antidepressants are so named due to the three rings of atoms that make up their basic structure.
- Atypical antidepressants are a group of drugs that do not easily fit into the first three categories.
- Monoamine Oxidase Inhibitors (MAOI's) stop enzymes within the body breaking down serotonin, dopamine and norepinephrine.

An interesting aspect of these drugs is, as a general rule, that improvement of depressive symptoms does not occur immediately. It may take up to fourteen days after the drug therapy commenced for improvement to be seen and felt. It is recognised that during this period of fourteen days the risk of suicide is increased and has a higher probability of occurring. The reasoning for this is still being debated. It may be the frustration of the person desperate for the drugs to work and believing that they have not. In this belief that the new medication has failed expectations once again and this may push a person over the edge. Other suppositions are that the person who commences a course of antidepressant medicine actually begins to take more of an interest in their lives, as the drugs improve their condition, till one day they actually have enough motivation and energy to finally jump.

Whatever the reasoning the fourteen-day watch period should be observed regardless as to whether it is a pharmaceutical or herb. Likewise, if you are self-administering the herbs, it will not be until the fourteenth day that you will be able to ascertain if the herbs are working or not and possibly try a different combination.

Whilst the imbalances of these chemicals have been widely researched and accepted into the established treatment regimens for depression, a person who is on a regime of antidepressants may not receive the full benefit from these drugs if diet or inflammatory conditions etc have not been addressed as well.

Further to this, the functioning of the thyroid, and the imbalances associated with this gland and its hormones, has also been researched and considered a causative factor. The two hormones secreted by the thyroid are triiodothyronine, known as T3 and thyroxine known as T4. Both hormones can be synthetically manufactured into medicines and administered by themselves, or in conjunction with the other antidepressants that work on the neurotransmitter monoamines. The genetic link to depression may be clearer in this instance as a familial history of thyroid problems would be able to be argued.

For those of you who may have thyroid issues the herbs considered scientifically useful are split into two groups:

- Thyroid suppressants – Bugleweed, Lemon Balm, Gromwell, Rosemary, Sage
- Thyroid stimulants – Gotu Kola, Bladderwrack, Guggul, Ashwagandha

More unusual consequences arise as we look deeper into the physical changes or imbalances when affected by depression. One of these has long been attributed to depression but has only recently been shown to be a real symptom. Depression is associated with gloomy colours such as black, blue or grey. Recent research has shown that the depressive person experiences changes in the way they perceive colour, and science has shown that a reduction in the perception of the shades of colour is a measurable affliction. A study from the university of Freiburg shows that depressed patients cannot view black and white contrasts accurately. A study in *Biological Psychiatry* showed a dramatically lower retinal contrast gain in patients with depression than in healthy subjects even if the patients were taking antidepressants at the time. This reduced sensitivity to colour is all the stranger, as the section of the brain that processes sight is the occipital lobe at the rear of the brain. As a result, the monoamine theory for depression that focuses on serotonin, dopamine and norepinephrine assumes that the midbrain or the limbic system is where depression manifests, is only one part of the puzzle.

So now we have various organs of the body either being affected by or creating a state of depression. Furthermore, researchers have shown that the monoamine dopamine is essential for the rod cells in the eyes to be able to receive colours and hence the complexity of depression deepens. In addition, depressive people are drawn to dull monotone colours. A study conducted in 2016 showed results supporting the assumption that depressive people prefer the colours black and grey. Consequently, colour therapy has become a popular therapeutic choice in its treatment. It would be logical to assume that a reduction in the feeling of depression should ensue when surrounded by bright warm colours, red, orange, pink etc.

Of note also is the finding that the more you are depressed the less you are able to smell. Here again, the complexity of depression expands. The olfactory bulb in the brain sits within the midbrain region or limbic and therefore supports the monoamine imbalance theory. As a sufferer of depression transitions negatively from mild depression to major depressive disorder, their sense of smell reduces. This is also true as a potential indicator of the various dementia syndromes such as Parkinson's disease and Alzheimer's disease. Therefore, we begin to see a symptomatology that can be used in diagnosing depressive states. However, treatment may not be simple due to these symptoms having causative factors that are not linked, and as a result one medication may not be sufficient in ameliorating the depressive state.

Another confirmed cause of depression is inflammation. Various research papers discuss the association between the inflammatory responses in the body and the onset or worsening of the depressive state. Meningitis (inflammation of the protective layer surrounding the spinal cord and brain), or encephalitis (inflammation of cerebral tissue) would therefore elicit a depression in the sufferer, yet autoimmune disease, arthritis, rheumatoid arthritis, Crohn's disease, multiple sclerosis and even gluten intolerance have all been associated with depression as well. Further still, environmental factors may also create an increase in inflammatory incidents, particularly when we consider pollution, pollen allergies, poisoning, smoking and poor diet. Some antidepressants reduce inflammation in the body, yet it is clear that ongoing research is still needed.

The broad suite of antidepressants focuses on the monoamine levels in the body in certain circumstances. The benefits from them are however small or ineffective if the core structures of the brain are deficient. Should there be a lack of neurons to process or be triggered by these monoamines then higher levels of them would be of no use. As we age or more specifically enter into old age, our ability to produce new neurons (neurogenesis) reduces, and this may be a factor in late onset of depression in people over 50. However, once again the lack of neurons may be due to genetic factors or trauma to the brain arising from injury or disease. In order to create new neurons, we need to supply our bodies with the necessary nutrients. Needless to say, a diet lacking in these will exacerbate the depressive episodes. The good news is that research has shown that some, not all, herbs scattered in this book actually stimulate neurogenesis. One example is Melissa Officinalis.

On a recent front in the late 1990's regulators allowed researchers access to previously restricted drugs such as psilocybin, from specific mushrooms, and lysergic acid diethylamide better known as LSD. These two drugs and their application to depressive conditions have created enormous excitement amongst sufferers and therapists alike. However, to date they remain outside the access of the normal depression membership list.

The science so far, whilst still 'fuzzy', continues to uncover causes and symptoms unique to the depressive state. Hormonal imbalances, dietary considerations, inflammatory actions, tissue degeneration, environmental factors all play a part. It may be that addressing only one of these would not result in any improvement, and accordingly a regime of treatment would be the best prescription for the sufferer of depression. Yet there is one factor that no amount of medicine can cure, and that is age. Research has identified two periods in a person's life where they will be more susceptible to a depression event: adolescence and old age. Yet each period is influenced by disparate causative factors. It has been found that younger people are more affected by factors such as electromagnetic pollution, and older people by financial and health factors.

[1] E. I. Fried, 'Problematic assumptions have slowed down depression research: Why symptoms, not syndromes are the way forward,' Front. Psychol., vol. 6, no. MAR, pp. 1–11, 2015.
[2] N. Fekadu, W. Shibeshi, and E. Engidawork, 'Major Depressive Disorder: Pathophysiology and Clinical Management.,' J. Depress. Anxiety, vol. 06, no. 01, pp. 1–7, 2017.
[3] M. Shadrina, E. A. Bondarenko, and P. A. Slominsky, 'Genetics factors in major depression disease,' Front. Psychiatry, vol. 9, no. JUL, pp. 1–18, 2018.
[4] T. Ljungberg, E. Bondza, and C. Lethin, 'Evidence of the importance of dietary habits regarding depressive symptoms and depression,' Int. J. Environ. Res. Public Health, vol. 17, no. 5, pp. 1–18, 2020.
[5] S. Singh and N. Kapoor, 'Health Implications of Electromagnetic Fields, Mechanisms of Action, and Research Needs,' Adv. Biol., vol. 2014, pp. 1–24, 2014.
[6] Khan, 'Chronic stress leads to anxiety and depression,' Ann Psychiatry Ment Heal., vol. 4, no. 7, p. 1087, 2016.
[7] C. H. Lee and F. Giuliani, 'The Role of Inflammation in Depression and Fatigue,' Front. Immunol., vol. 10, no. July, p. 1696, 2019.
[8] 'NEUROSCIENCE - Scientific American Article on IQ and depression.'.
[9] R. Shah, A. Shah, and P. Links, 'Post-traumatic stress disorder and depression comorbidity: Severity across different populations,' Neuropsychiatry (London)., vol. 2, no. 6, pp. 521–529, 2012.
[10] N. Surgery, 'Imported from http://ijomeh.eu/Impact-of-air-pollution-on-depression-and-suicide-a-review-article-,84931,0,2.html,' vol. 31, no. 6, pp. 711–721, 2018.
[11] G. M. Goodwin, 'Depression and associated physical diseases and symptoms,' Dialogues Clin. Neurosci., vol. 8, no. 2, pp. 259–265, 2006.
[12] S. M. A. Dijkstra-Kersten, K. E. M. Biesheuvel-Leliefeld, J. C. van der Wouden, B. W. J. H. Penninx, and H. W. J. van Marwijk, 'Associations of financial strain and income with depressive and anxiety disorders,' J. Epidemiol. Community Health, vol. 69, no. 7, pp. 660–665, 2015.
[13] B. M. Street, 'The relationship between age and depression: a self-efficacy model,' 2004.
[14] A. Akin and M. İskender, 'Internet Addiction and Depression, Anxiety and Stress,' Int. Online J. Educ. Sci., vol. 3, no. 1, pp. 138–148, 2011.
[15] L. Walsh, 'Causes of Depression,' Depress. Care across Lifesp., pp. 1–17, 2010.
[16] M. Hinz, A. Stein, and T. Uncini, 'The discrediting of the monoamine hypothesis,' Int. J. Gen. Med., vol. 5, pp. 135–142, 2012.
[17] M. P. Hage and S. T. Azar, 'The link between thyroid function and depression,' J. Thyroid Res., vol. 2012, no. January 2012, 2012.
[18] D. K. Chanchal, A. Gupta, W. Suchita, and G. Bina, 'Herbal Drugs for Thyroid,' Int. J. Pharm. Biol. Sci., vol. 6, no. 1, pp. 62–70, 2016.
[19] E. Bubl, L. Tebartz Van Elst, M. Gondan, D. Ebert, and M. W. Greenlee, 'Vision in depressive disorder,' World J. Biol. Psychiatry, vol. 10, no. 4 PART 2, pp. 377–384, 2009.
[20] S. Korkmaz, Ö. Özer, Ş. Kaya, A. Kazgan, and M. Atmaca, 'The correlation between color choices and impulsivity, anxiety and depression,' Eur. J. Gen. Med., vol. 13, no. 3, pp. 47–50, 2016.

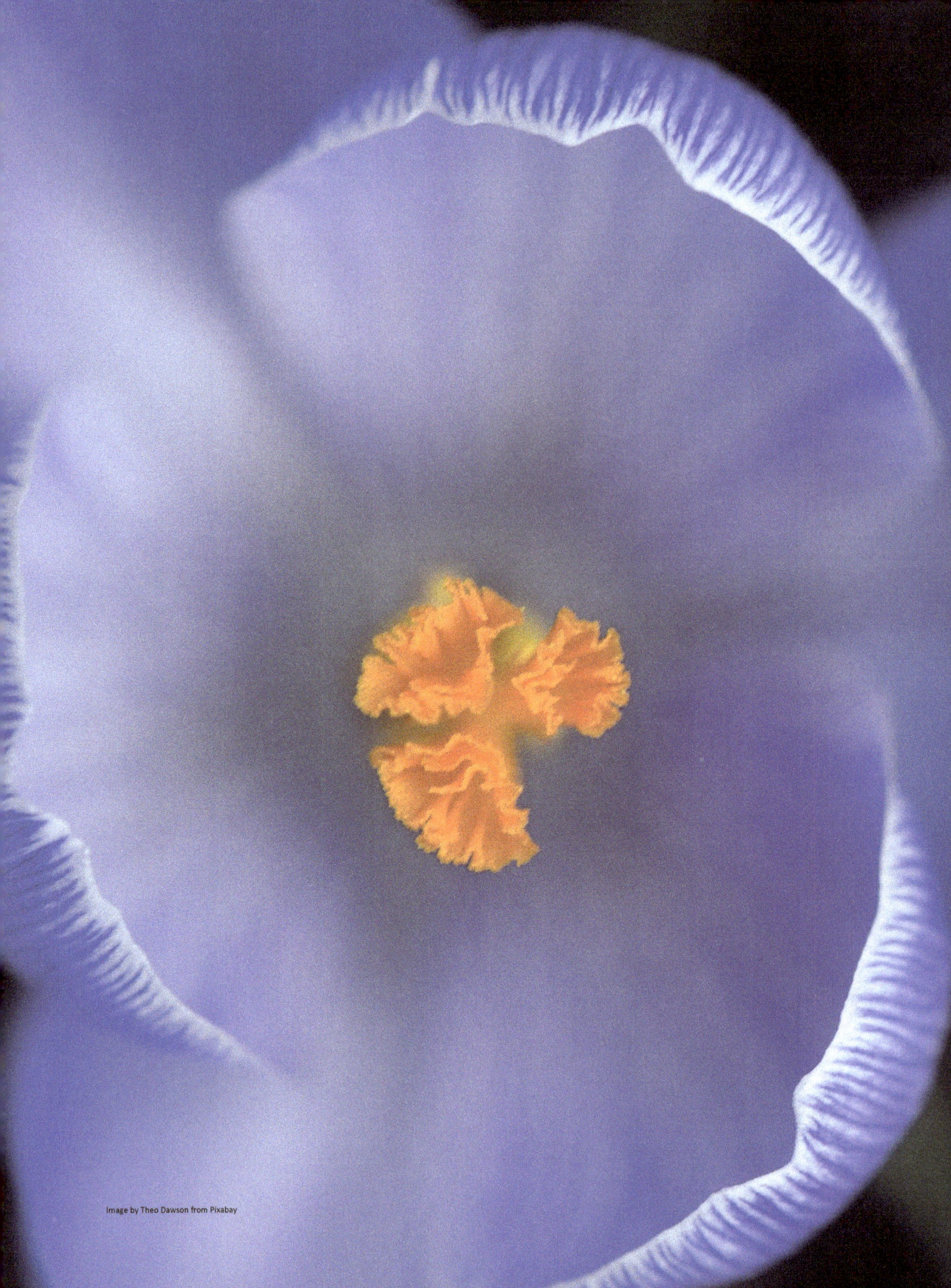
Image by Theo Dawson from Pixabay

Saffron - Crocus sativus

The history of Saffron is fascinating. There are claims that it has been found in prehistoric rock art paintings dating back 50,000 years. What we know for sure is that people have been using Saffron for a long time and that Crocus has been cultivated intentionally for approximately 3,500 years. The origin of Saffron is not known, but some suspect the birthplace to be the area of modern-day Iran. Regardless of where Crocus sativus originated it is grown all over the world primarily due to it being the most expensive herb or spice on the planet.

The reason behind the price of the herb is that it takes an estimated 180,000 flowers to make just one kilo of Saffron. Only the three small stigmas found in the flowers are used and these have to be gently picked by hand. As a result, one kilogram of Saffron may cost anywhere from $1,000 to $10,000 making it more expensive than gold. Fortunately, research has found that the petals of the flowers also act medicinally in much the same way as the spice.

It is believed that the main compounds found in the stigmas, safranal, crocin, crocetin and picrocrocin, make the herb such an effective antidepressant. Some of the compounds found in the stigmas give them the unique yellow-red colouring, yet the petals are a light purple and also act as an antidepressant.

In various studies, the saffron spice has been compared to several standard antidepressants, two of which have been imipramine and fluoxetine. The results have shown that both its stigmas and petals of the flowers displayed similar properties as the two standard drugs. A 2018 review on scientific trials into the effects of saffron for depression discussed the neuron protecting effects of the herb as well as the suspected influence on serotonin, dopamine and norepinephrine amines. Not only was it found that Crocus sativus acts as an antidepressant, it also protects memory and cognitive function, making it an ideal herb for degenerative diseases of the brain in later life.

Testing of the herb on depression with doses ranging from 200 mg-800 mg per kilo bodyweight for the stigmas from the flower and 300 mg per kilo bodyweight for its petals showed them to be highly effective in treating mild to moderate depression, over a six-week period.

Whilst it has been shown that the use of Crocus sativus is relatively safe and that it has minimal side effects, the research has also shown that the herb should not be taken by pregnant women because it produces birth defects and even termination of pregnancy in animal studies. Other than this caution, the herb has been shown to be relatively nontoxic up to 2000 gm to bodyweight dose. Other research has found that long term use of Saffron may lower blood pressure, body temperature, and due to its antiplatelet actions, it can promote bleeding. As a result, in the right circumstances, the above list of side effects may be desirable in someone suffering from high blood pressure and other cardiac challenges, but they might not be desirable for someone with low blood pressure.

[1] Yang XY, Chen XL, Fu YX, Luo QH, Du L, Qiu HT, Qiu T, Zhang L, Meng HQ. Comparative efficacy and safety of Crocus sativus L. for treating mild to moderate major depressive disorder in adults: a meta-analysis of randomized controlled trials. *Neuropsychiatr Dis Treat*. 2018;14:1297-1305

[2] B.Poojar et al. "Methodology used in the study" Asian J. Pharm. Clin. Res. Vol 7, no 10, pp 1-5, 2017

[3] "Crocus Sativus Saffron PFAF Database.

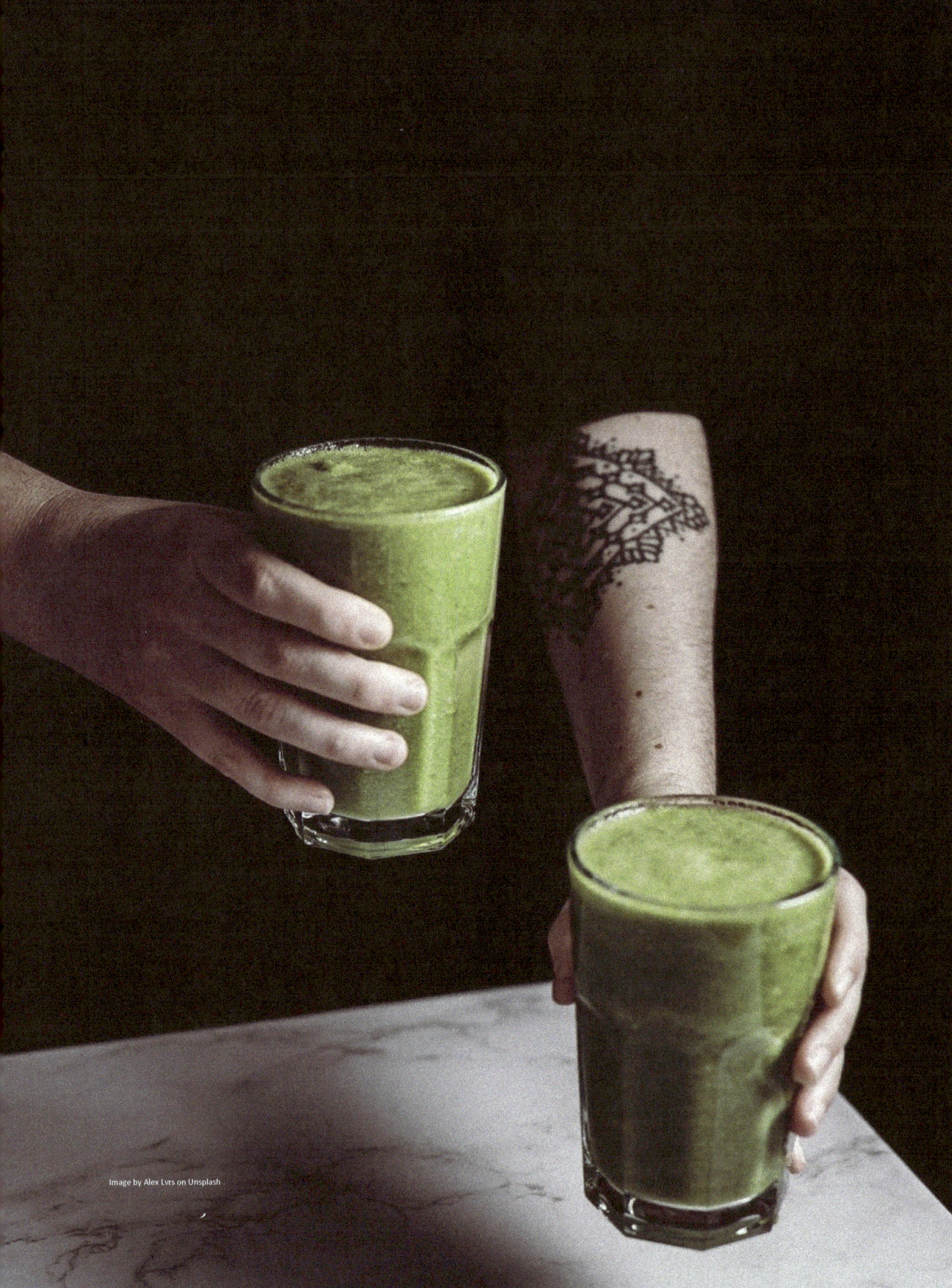

Image by Alex Lvrs on Unsplash

Celery - Apium graveolens

When the internet heats up with viral trends of the latests and greatests, we tend to ignore it because much could simply be nonsense. However, in the study of our vegetable celery, it becomes a welcome surprise to find that the hype is well deserved.

Celery has been around for a very long time. It is reported that there are pictures of celery flowers in Tutankhamun's tomb, and in the temple complex devoted to Hera on the island of Samos celery seeds were found that date back to the seventh century BC. So, this staple kitchen vegetable has a long and venerable history. In ancient northern Greece its leaves and flowers were associated with death, and was believed to have originated from the blood of one of the ancient Gods of the Cabeiri, a cult from the islands surrounding Lemnos in the Aegean Sea. The use of celery as a medicine has been found in both Unani and Ayurvedic health systems dating back well before Christ.

Throughout the historical use of celery, it was not merely used as a food but also as an important medicinal plant. Various health claims have been made, some of which dealt with cardioprotective as well as anticancer.

It comes as no surprise that we now find an enormous amount of research applied to its benefits. One such paper (2012) resulted in the finding that a dose of 200 mg/kg of the methanolic extract made from celery seeds was as effective as the tricyclic antidepressant imipramine. As imipramine is also used for panic attacks and anxiety, it may be safe to assume that celery seed extract may be as effective for these two conditions as well. The research (2012) has been cited in many other papers on the benefits of this herb. Additionally, a report from 2016 from Thailand, delved deeper into the antidepressant effects of an extract made from the entire plant. It found that not only did the extract reduce depression significantly, but it also increased cognitive functions such as memory and learning. When compared to the standard drug for dementia, donepezil, the celery extract was as effective. This study found that celery extract compared favourably when assessed with the standard anti-depression drug fluoxetine.

The oil made from its seeds is high in selinene, a compound thought to be responsible for the antidepressant action. However, another compound known as apigenin is found in both celery and chamomile, and as we all know, chamomile has a reputation as a relaxant. So, the orchestra of organic chemistry is once more at play here. It may be a combination of chemical compounds found in its seeds that are working synergistically to bring about positive changes in people suffering from depression.

The use of celery juice and extract has been studied in a wide range of health conditions with many positive results for cardiac support, liver protection, antibacterial, antifungal and also weight loss. While all this sounds exciting, caution should be used as we are all different. A person who suffers from low blood pressure may consider the use of celery not ideal, and likewise for other health conditions such as gastrointestinal problems that may be exacerbated by its use.

Some people are highly allergic to celery; a simple test of rubbing the juice from the plant on the sensitive skin under the wrist will show a reaction of a red rash if you are.

[1] N. Anwar, N. Z. Ahmed, T. Shahida, K. Kabiruddin, and H. Aslam, "The Role of Mufarrehat (Exhilarants) in the Management of Depression: An Evidence Based Approach," J. Psychiatry, vol. 20, no. 5, 2017.

[2] N. Saini, G. K. Singh, and B. P. Nagori, "Spasmolytic potential of some medicinal plants belonging to family umbelliferae: A review," Int. J. Res. Ayurveda Pharm., vol. 5, no. 1, pp. 74–83, 2014.

[3] P. Boonruamkaew et al., "Apium graveolens extract influences mood and cognition in healthy mice," J. Nat. Med., vol. 71, no. 3, pp. 492–505, 2017.

[4] Brahma Srinivasa Rao Desu and Sivaramakrishna K, "Anti-Depressant Activity of Methanolic Extract of Apium Graveolens Seeds," Int. J. Res. Pharm. Chem., vol. 2, no. 4, pp. 1124–1127, 2012.

[5] P. D. A. E. Al-Snafi, "Medicinal plants with central nervous effects (part 2): plant based review," IOSR J. Pharm., vol. 06, no. 08, pp. 52–75, 2016.

[6] A. E. Al-snafi, "International Journal for Pharmaceutical Research Scholars (IJPRS)," no. January 2014, pp. 671–677, 2014.

Why herbs

"The whole problem with the world is that fools and fanatics are always so certain of themselves, and wiser people so full of doubts"

Bertrand Russell

It is estimated that over 80 per cent of the world's underprivileged developing population relies on traditional medicinal systems in order to cure sickness and improve health. Should this statistic be correct, and there is no reason to doubt it as it is cited in many research papers, then the resulting reliance on traditional medicine in the form of herbs is the only avenue of health care for possibly 4 billion people.

Sadly, a surviving significant portion of these traditional health systems are ineffective. Many of these systems are still being studied and verified with impressive results, yet in some cases, traditional cures have been found to have no effect at all. On the other hand, the negative results can also be regarded as positives, because they can now stop people trusting ineffective and even dangerous therapies from unnecessary pain or disease with the scientific research now confirming or denying their effective properties.

Throughout history nature supplied people with unique solutions for food, shelter, and medicine, but only in the last 150 years has medicine been transformed, through science and chemistry, to now be able to make synthetic drugs that are more precise and effective in the treatment of disease. Yet, whilst the potency of these new drugs cannot be denied, the serious and more powerful side effects cannot be ignored either. In the field of antidepressant drugs this is well understood and grudgingly tolerated due to the undeniable improvement many people experience via their use.

People have sought remedies from nature for thousands of years. Much of the herbal or traditional systems have evolved from trial and error and have been refined over time into systems such as the Ayurvedic, Unani, American Indian, Aboriginal, and countless others, all unique to the environments in which the people lived. In recent times modern scientific research has re-examined these systems and the plants within them, seeking new and more effective drugs and treatments. Such research, for the most part was instigated with the aim of discovering unique alkaloids or compounds that could be refined and standardised into pharmaceutical drugs. It has now been reported that as much as 50% and possibly 75% of over-the-counter drugs on the market nowadays are either sourced directly from plants or contain some form of botanically derived principle. In addition, there is an emerging middle ground of people becoming more interested in using the pure plant in its entirety rather than a pharmaceutical drug. This 'retro' acceptance and demand for more holistic treatments are being driven by two influences, cost and fear of drug dependency.

In the developed world more and more people are seeking solutions from traditional medicine and their herbal extracts, powders or tisanes. In America it was reported that the growth of the herbal medicine market was increasing at a rate of 30% annually, with the predominant user having a high-school education or higher, hence indicating that the consumer is either open to new therapies, or that they understand their health needs, or both.

In the developed world Germany stands out as one of Europe's largest importers of herbal medicines with approximately 45,000 tons of raw herbal medicines imported annually. China has long employed two systems of medicine, with one being the traditional system and the other modern medicine. In so doing, they have successfully bonded the medicinal systems as 'complementary' to each other. In 2018, the global herbal supplement market had an estimated value of 99.9 billion US dollars and an expectation to grow by 8% per annum to reach 171 billion US dollars in 2025. Naturally, where significant financial gain is to be had, one can expect sub-standard products, false claims, and fraudulent practices. Nonetheless, demand continues to grow, and this is a key piece of evidence in the overall argument of the effectiveness of the plants.

Needless to say, as with all discussions proponents for and against exist. Those that believe herbal medicines are ineffective and even dangerous, and those that argue to the counter. Despite this debate, a clear and logical view should be to accept herbal medicines once they have been properly and rigorously studied and verified.

Whilst we do not consider everyday items in our lives as herbal, they are undeniably so. Our coffee in the morning is in fact an herbal tisane, which we use as a morning stimulant. An afternoon or evening beer is a common choice with its medieval blend of hops, malted barley and yeast. Hops (*Humulus lupus*) is a member of the Hemp family (*Cannabaceae*) and is used as a sedative and relaxant. Yet Hops is also one of the best sources of oestrogen and is used in hormone replacement therapy for menopausal women. Ginger has a long and well-studied use as a treatment for nausea and cramps. These, and many more plants in our everyday diets have countless scientific papers written on them supporting the health claims, such as vincristine from the periwinkle plant. Nevertheless, there will always be doubters or worse, experts who dismiss herbal medicines as ill-informed witchcraft and quackery. Regardless, in our hospitals and medical clinics morphine, atropine, artemisinin, digitalis, paclitaxel, aspirin, quinine and other drugs are directly sourced from plants. Aspirin, its natural derivative, as an example is sourced from the bark of the Willow tree. The constant denial of the effectiveness of herbal medicines is therefore disingenuous, to say the least. There remain challenges however with prescribing the most effective dosage of the herbal preparations as there are variations in the level of active compounds within the plants, even in the same species. This is mainly due to soil conditions or production variations, such as when a plant is grown in a foreign climatic zone, undergoes variations in the weather patterns from one harvest to the next (rainfall or lack thereof), and simply genetic variations in a population. As a result, achieving a precise repeatable dose for any herbal supplement is almost impossible. The pharmaceutical medicine however can be extremely precise in the prescribed dosage.

For the remote areas of our planet, it would be unconscionable to deny any form of comfort due to this bigotry and bias, on both sides as to whether herbal medicines are or are not a solution. In 2017, more children died from dysentery than almost any other early childhood disease. The treatment for dysentery however is cheap and effective, yet almost impossible to deliver to Central Africa and other areas of the world trapped in perennial wars, corruption, or distance. For dysentery it has been shown that the common herb thyme is highly effective in the control of gastrointestinal issues caused by pathogens. A possible solution for these isolated communities would be education and seeds of the effective plant.

Depression has many levels of clinical diagnosis, from mild to acute, from Seasonal Affected Disorder (SAD) to Major Depressive Disorder (MDD) and everything in between. The symptoms of depression vary too and can be vague and uncertain. These range from lack of appetite, lack of energy, weight gain to thoughts of suicide. Therefore, we can clearly agree that there is still a great deal of misunderstanding and confusion surrounding depression and its causes. As a result, the ethical therapist would welcome any tool or strategy to help their patients improve with the lowest potential for side effects and harm.

Herbal medicines are not, nor should, ever counter the modern scientific medical practices that our hospitals, doctors and therapists employ every day. Rather they should be a soft and less intrusive option for the commencement of therapy or be complementary as in many cases, patients may not have enough improvement from herbs alone and then the pharmaceutical drugs can be introduced in conjunction with or replacing the herbal preparation.

The level of the world's population expected to suffer from depression and anxiety is modelled to rise over time. The reasons for this epidemic are still being debated, yet such discussions offer little comfort to the sufferers today.

I advocate with this book that it is remarkably simple to grow a plant, and it is only somewhat more complex to make herbal preparations.

[1] Q. Liu, H. He, J. Yang, X. Feng, F. Zhao, and J. Lyu, "Changes in the global burden of depression from 1990 to 2017: Findings from the Global Burden of Disease study," *J. Psychiatr. Res.*, vol. 126, no. August 2019, pp. 134–140, 2019.

[2] N. Tagalidou, E. Distlberger, V. Loderer, and A. R. Laireiter, "Efficacy and feasibility of a humor training for people suffering from depression, anxiety, and adjustment disorder: A randomized controlled trial," *BMC Psychiatry*, vol. 19, no. 1, pp. 1–13, 2019.

[3] U. Willinger *et al.*, "Cognitive and emotional demands of black humour processing: the role of intelligence, aggressiveness and mood," *Cogn. Process.*, vol. 18, no. 2, pp. 159–167, 2017.

[4] 北村純一 *et al.*, "1. 顔面麻痺タイプの診断に難渋した1症例 (第1回 日本リハビリテーション医学会関東地方会)," *Japanese J. Rehabil. Med.*, vol. 34, no. 3, pp. 234–235, 1997.

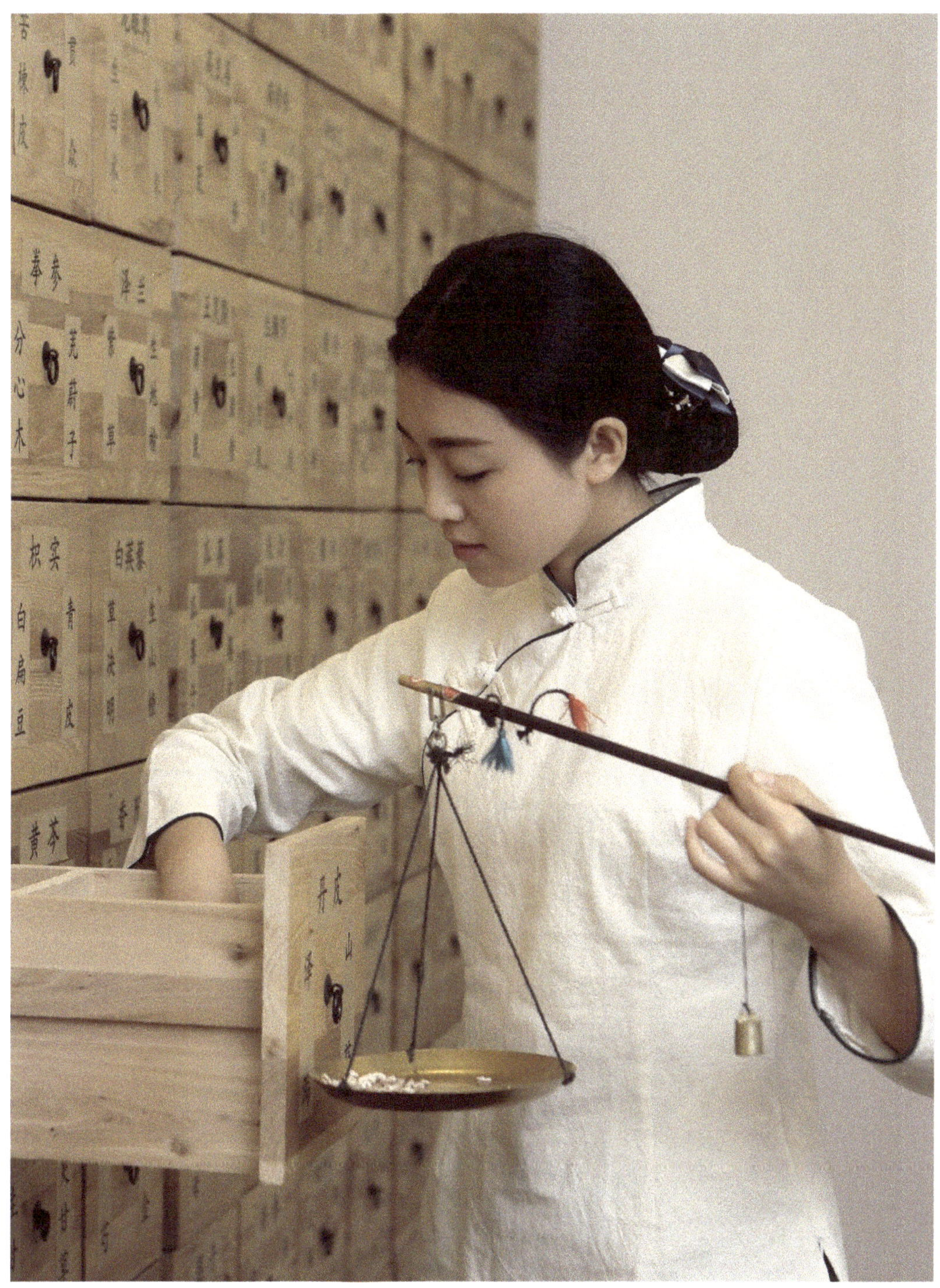

Image by kian2018 from Pixabay

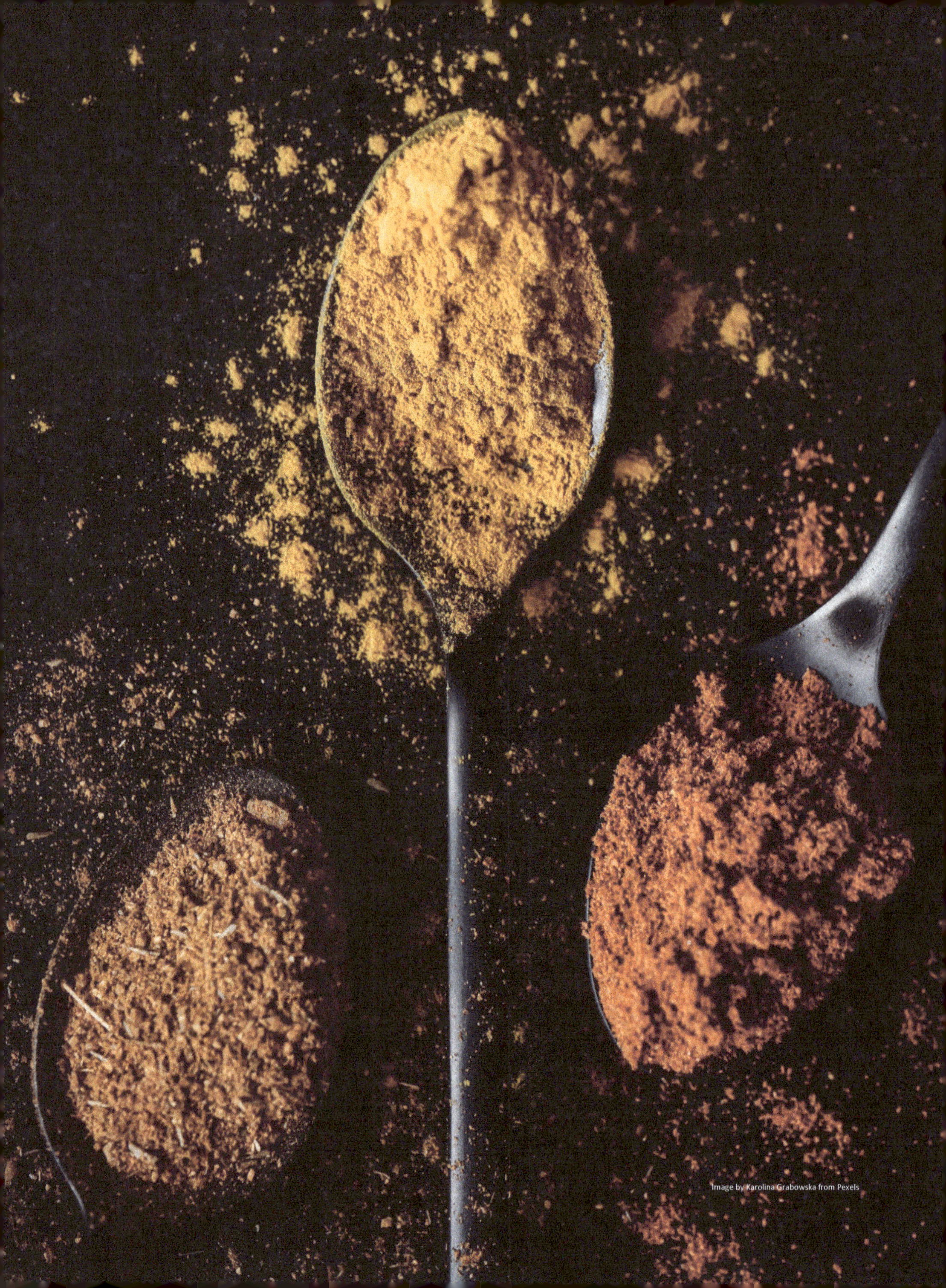

Image by Karolina Grabowska from Pexels

Turmeric - Curcuma longa

If there was to be a diva of the alternative health world, then Turmeric would surely be it. There are so many claims about this colourful root that you would not be mistaken in thinking that it can cure almost anything. Sadly, this is not the case. Yet the root of the plant is useful in various health complaints, and as a result it has been in use for centuries in Ayurvedic, Unani and Chinese medicine. Turmeric is a relative of the well-known ginger plant.

In character with scientific research, there are claims and counterclaims as to the efficacy of turmeric. However, as the plant is entirely non-toxic it will not do you any harm. If you feel it is helping you in any way, then you can disregard the negative results from the various clinical trials that are anti the herb.

A great deal of scientific focus has been on the compound known as curcumin derived from the root of Curcuma longa. This unique compound is further described as diferuloyl methane and is thought to be responsible for many of the health claims associated with the plant. A paper (2015), jointly undertaken by researchers in both Taiwan and Japan, showed that curcumin did indeed positively influence depressive symptomology and had similar effects as that of the standard drug imipramine.

As far back as 2002 the research from the Institute of Functional Biomolecule, State Key Laboratory of Pharmaceutical Biotechnology, School of Life Sciences, Nanjing university, Nanjing, China also showed strong results in the use of the whole root extract in the alleviation of depression. In this paper, the researchers arrived at the conclusion that doses of 560 mg/kg body weight had a more effective benefit than fluoxetine, and the extract further reduced monoamine oxidase in the tissue of the laboratory animals. The monoamine oxidase group of compounds reduce the time that neurotransmitters such as serotonin, dopamine and norepinephrine are active, and as a result are thought to reduce feelings of wellbeing in people suffering from depression.

Another well-known action of curcumin is its anti-inflammatory ability. This has been researched and established since the early 1990s. Here again it is seen that inflammation and the reduction of it have been linked to improvement in depressive states.

A further paper, completed in 2014, discussed the effects of curcumin and other curcuminoids found in its root on the activity of specific regions of the brain associated with mood and behaviour. This article discussed the various neuronal actions of curcumin and found that the compound has significant and measurable actions on nerve function and health. The researchers found that curcumin protected the frontal cortex, hypothalamus and hippocampus regions of the brain from stress induced responses as well as reducing glutamate actions in the regulation of monoamine neurotransmitter function.

Curcuma longa has been used to treat other conditions such as a cardiac tonic, antithrombotic, anti-arthritic, hypoglycaemic, liver tonic and anticancer.

[1] H. Collaborator, "Name of dispatched researcher Af À liation of Instructor Host Collaborator," no. 6.

[2] P. P. S, S. P. Roy, N. Patel, and K. J. Gohil, "RESEARCH AND REVIEWS: JOURNAL OF PHARMACOGNSOY AND PHYTOCHEMISTRY Curcumin as an Antidepressant: A Review .," vol. 2, no. 2, pp. 29–34, 2014.

[3] S. K. Kulkarni, A. Dhir, and K. K. Akula, "Potentials of curcumin as an antidepressant," Scientific World Journal., vol. 9, no. 2009, pp. 1233–1241, 2009.

[4] Z. F. Yu, L. D. Kong, and Y. Chen, "Antidepressant activity of aqueous extracts of Curcuma longa in mice," J. Ethnopharmacol., vol. 83, no. 1–2, pp. 161–165, 2002.

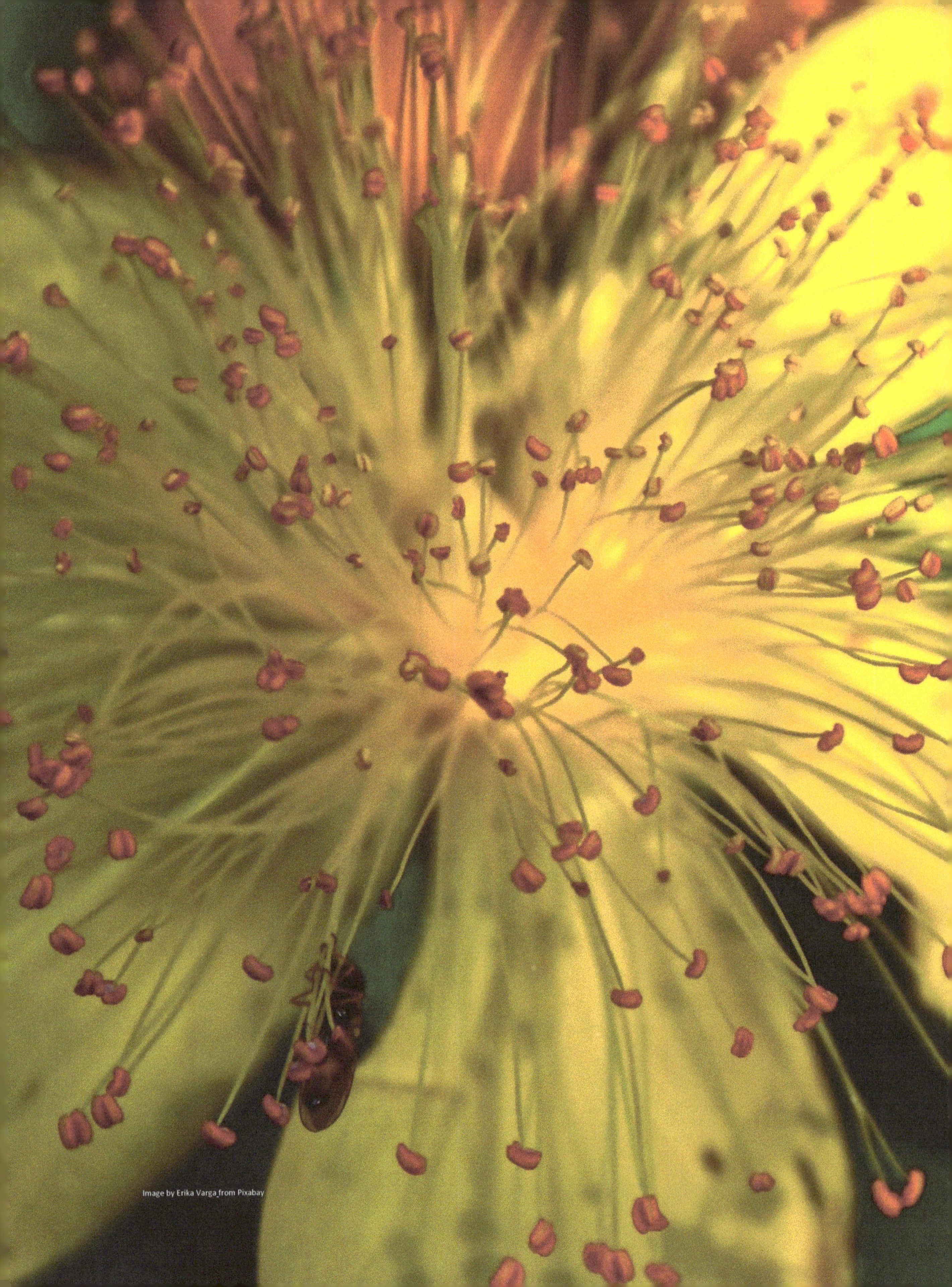

Image by Erika Varga from Pixabay

St John's Wort - Hypericum perforatum

If there were to be a superstar of the herbal treatments for depression, then St John's Wort would be it. It is sold across the world in both pill and extract form specifically for depression relief. However, just like a superstar, it has its bad boy side and should be well understood before you decide to take it.

St John's Wort has been used for thousands of years, and famously it was the herb of choice for the Order of St John as an antibiotic in treating the wounds of knights during the crusades. We may safely assume this is where it obtained its common name. Yet, the flowers bloom each year in Europe around the summer solstice in late June and which is also when St John's Day is celebrated. It was common for the flowers to be hung over doorways and above religious icons during this time, which may explain its scientific name of Hypericum which means 'hung above' in Latin.

The two main compounds found in the herb, hyperforin and hypericin, are thought to be responsible for the antidepressant actions. In a meta-analysis of 37 papers on the antidepressant effects of St John's Wort in 2005, the authors found that there were significant inconsistencies in results, and that the effects of the herb in more robust studies were minor only for people suffering from chronic depression. The real support for the herb is to be found in the adverse effects of the plant use. St John's Wort causes adverse complications when used in conjunction with some standard drugs used to treat depression, especially serotonin reuptake inhibitors. Serotonin Syndrome can occur, which is a surplus of serotonin in the blood, causing agitation, confusion, high temperatures, dilated pupils, tremors, sweating and diarrhoea. As a result, the herb should not be used by people taking other medications for depression, heart conditions, cancer medications, HIV medications and anti-coagulants. Pregnant women should definitely not use the herb as it may abort the child. On the upside, it confirms that St John's Wort affects the monoamine regulators, otherwise such side effects would not occur. As they say, "Thou do protest too much Sir!" all the negative claims about the herb are in effect the best evidence for its use.

We can see from the complications that the herb shows its 'bad boy side', yet it has been highly effective for many people who suffer from mild depression. User's discretion is recommended.

The other health aspects of St John's Wort that have been studied in various trials are its antiviral, antibiotic, diuretic and wound healing actions, all of which have been supported to a greater or lesser extent.

The native range for growing Hypericum perforatum was temperate Europe and Asia, however it has now been introduced across the globe, and is even considered to be an invasive weed. A reputation due to its out-competing native grasses and vegetation, as it replaces fodder sources for ruminants such as cows, horses, and sheep. Because the herb is toxic to these animals, with symptoms experienced that are very similar to Serotonin Syndrome, it has become a significant challenge for farmers.

[1] T. Mennini and M. Gobbi, "The antidepressant mechanism of Hypericum perforatum," Life Sci., vol. 75, no. 9, pp. 1021–1027, 2004.

[2] K. Linde, M. Berner, M. Egger, and C. Mulrow, "St John's wort for depression: Meta-analysis of randomised controlled trials," Br. J. Psychiatry, vol. 186, no. FEB., pp. 99–107, 2005.

[3] J. Tian, F. Zhang, J. Cheng, S. Guo, P. Liu, and H. Wang, "Antidepressant-like activity of adhyperforin, a novel constituent of Hypericum perforatum L.," Sci. Rep., vol. 4, pp. 1–6, 2014.

[4] Committee on Herbal Medicinal Products (HMPC), "Assessment report on Hypericum perforatum," Eur. Med. agency Eval. Med. Hum. Use, vol. 44, no. November, pp. 1–77, 2009.

[5] A. Nahrstedt, "Antidepressant Constituents of Hypericum perforatum," no. January 2000, pp. 144–153, 1997.

It's all too funny

"To truly laugh, you must be able to take your pain, and play with it"

Charlie Chaplin

Research has sought to understand the link between comedy and depression with varying degrees of clarity and understanding. It is the strange ability of a person to see humour even though they are crippled with anxiety and fear. Most sufferers of depression possess a wry and cynical view of themselves possibly due to an overactive pursuit of self-analysis and self-loathing being hidden under a dark veneer of humour and jokes. Comedy is the perfect camouflage for the depressed, as Rodney Dangerfield, a famous American comedian liked to say.

Sigmund Freud, the father of psychoanalysis, stated that "comedians often tell jokes as a kind of relief system for some kind of anxiety". The shock and surprise audiences have when a famous comedian takes his or her life is proportional to the perception of their fame as a comedian. Statements like "But he/she was so funny!" indicate society's belief that funny people should be happy all the time due to their ability to make people laugh. Yet it appears to be the exact opposite. Case in point is the passing of actor and comedian Robin Williams.

Depressed people view the world as a confusing and cruel place. They spend a great deal of time not simply analysing themselves but also their place in society and why they don't fit in. Their analysis questions all aspects of life and more often than not encounters aspects that are full of paradox, irony and contradiction, and which in turn produces a wealth of material for comedians. As Mark Twain said, "The secret source of humour is not joy, but sorrow. There is no humour in heaven." Therefore, it is assumed that the great bulk of comedy originates from emotional and physical pain. Slapstick comedy is a clear example of this as it strives to entertain audiences with a primary figure experiencing all manner of humiliation and tragedy. Nonetheless, research over the past decades has not discovered a definitive correlation between depression and comedy.

Recent studies into the use of humour as a therapy to alleviate symptoms of depression have also arrived at an impasse, where the belief that humour is effective as a therapeutic medium is supported even when findings do not correlate with this belief. In much of the research, it was found that humour did alleviate depressive-like symptoms but for only short periods of time. The comedian George Carlin might have summed this up in his quote "Fighting for peace is like fucking for virginity!" As humour appears to be the creation of depression, using it to alleviate it appears to be destined to fail.

In 2005, the Times newspaper conducted a test on 12 comedians from the Edinburgh Fringe Festival and found overwhelming evidence that in order to be good at comedy you had to have an above average IQ. In this test, the comedians were asked to undertake the MENSA IQ test from the oldest and largest high IQ society in the world. Four of the comedians immediately gained entry into the MENSA society and another three were borderline. In another research paper it was shown that black humour or black comedy, also known as dark comedy, dark humour or gallows humour, is a comic style that makes light of subject matter that is generally considered taboo. Particularly the subjects that are normally considered serious or too painful to discuss required above average intelligence. In this study, 156 candidates were shown dark humour cartoons. Those with a high level of appreciation for such humour had high non-verbal and verbal intelligence. Here we start to see the correlation between depression and humour, in so much as the type of comedy becomes an important factor. Other types of comedy are romantic comedy, blue comedy (sexual), political satire and screwball comedy (bizarre), yet all genres are recognised as blending into each other to some extent. More specifically comedians who are self-deprecating have been found to have a higher ratio of depression. This elevation of making fun of yourself into a comedy skit would be in keeping with what people suffering from low self-esteem do naturally. As one of my dearest life-long friends said to me once "If it weren't for bad luck, I would have no luck at all". A study conducted in Staffordshire England investigated humour in school children and is quoted in a BBC report as showing clear evidence that children who are bullied, use self-defeating humour to placate children who seek to bully them. This humour, the report states, is maladaptive and gives rise to low self-esteem later in life.

A result of all of this has been volumes of research into the links, either positive or negative, of humour being associated with depression and despair. It seems that the sad clown complex as it has come to be called is part of the symptomology of depression and that the comedian that you are laughing at may actually be desperately in need of help and not your laughter.

Depressive people will use various tactics or methods to hide their inner demons from the prying eyes of others, and witty humour is one of them. Perhaps it stems from the desire to be liked, and the fear that should people learn of the confusion and internal self-loathing they will not be liked as much or enough. There is one thing that people with depression definitely don't want and that is pity. Pity is poison to the depressed, as by its very nature it assumes a higher position or condescending attitude that verifies all the negative thoughts in the sad clown's head. The act of feeling sorry for someone or pitying them solidifies a relationship of superior to inferior. Hence, the use of humour to ensure this aspect never happens.

No matter the subtleties of the scientific literature and endless debates into humour and depression, if you are one of these people who is the life of the party and use self-critical or defeating humour, then you may very well be depressed. Conversely, if you know someone who is like this then perhaps you don't really know them at all.

You may like to ask whether your black dog enjoys a good laugh from time to time.

[1] [Q. Liu, H. He, J. Yang, X. Feng, F. Zhao, and J. Lyu, "Changes in the global burden of depression from 1990 to 2017: Findings from the Global Burden of Disease study," J. Psychiatr. Res., vol. 126, no. August 2019, pp. 134–140, 2019.

[2] N. Tagalidou, E. Distlberger, V. Loderer, and A. R. Laireiter, "Efficacy and feasibility of a humor training for people suffering from depression, anxiety, and adjustment disorder: A randomized controlled trial," BMC Psychiatry, vol. 19, no. 1, pp. 1–13, 2019.

[3] U. Willinger et al., "Cognitive and emotional demands of black humour processing: the role of intelligence, aggressiveness and mood," Cogn. Process., vol. 18, no. 2, pp. 159–167, 2017.

[4] 北村純一 et al., "1. 顔面麻痺タイプの診断に難渋した1症例 (第1回 日本リハビリテーション医学会関東地方会)," Japanese J. Rehabil. Med., vol. 34, no. 3, pp. 234–235, 1997.

[5] Danzer A, Dale JA, Klions AHL. Effect of Exposure to Humorous Stimuli on Induced Depression. Psychological Reports. 1990;66(3):1027-1036. doi:10.2466/pr0.1990.66.3.1027.

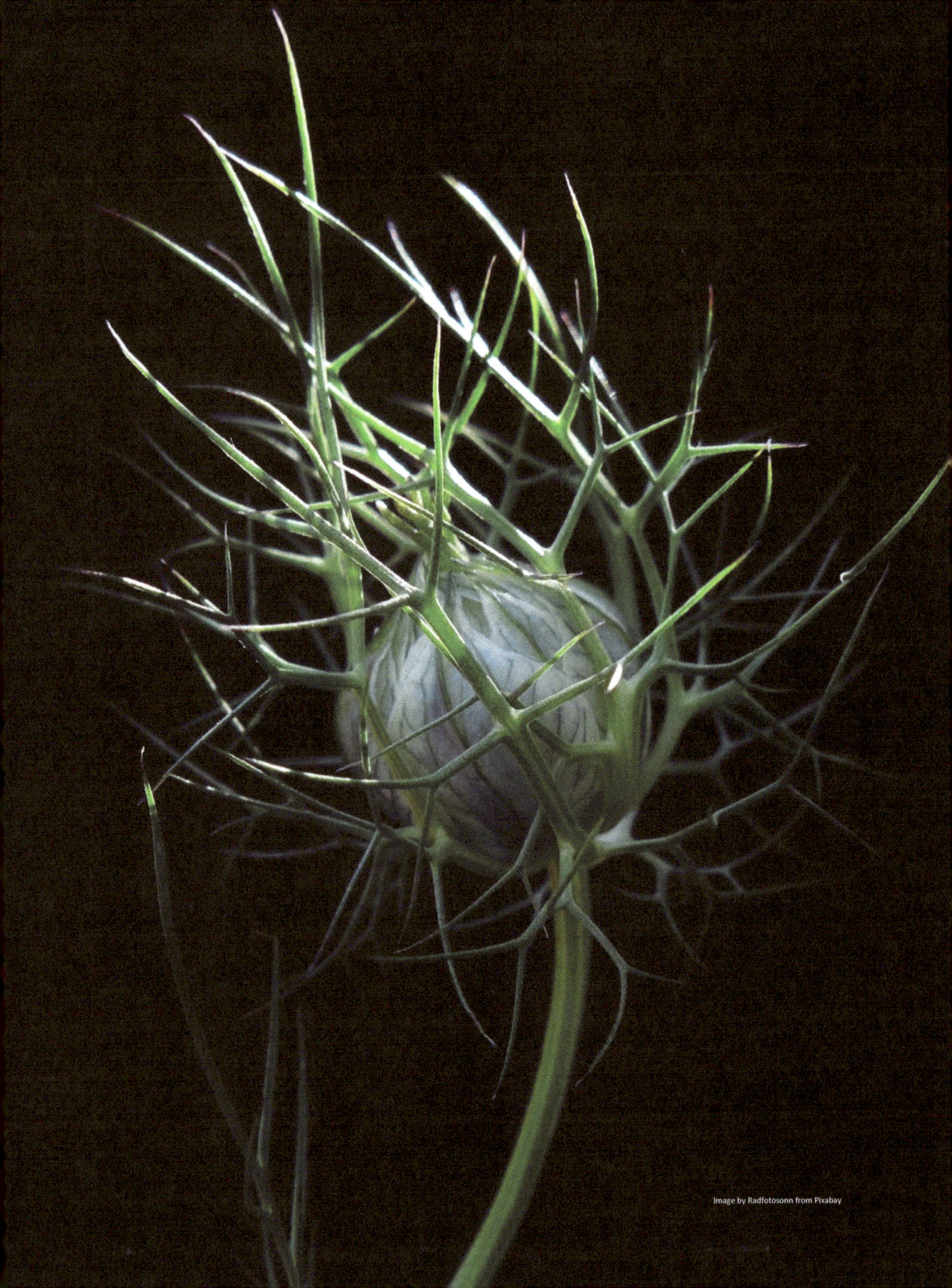

Image by Radfotosonn from Pixabay

Cumin - Cuminum cynimum

Once again, a member of the Apiaceae genus of plants or more commonly known as the parsley family. Cumin has been used for thousands of years and is thought to have originated from the eastern Mediterranean. It is now used worldwide as a food spice and flavour enhancer. Yet, it is the medicinal attributes of the plant that make it truly unique.

A great deal of research has been conducted on the various health claims associated with Cumin, and with the majority of this research being undertaken in the last decade or so. Research from 2001 showed that the essential oil from the fruits of the plant significantly improved memory and helped in the reversal of amnesia. As a result, it is understood that Cumin has a positive tonic-like effect on the limbic system within the brain where we store our memories and emotions.

Another aspect of the use of Cumin is the anti-inflammatory actions of the plant. It has been shown in separate studies that the essential oil from the plant reduced oxidative stress in the body, and in doing so may have neuroprotective actions of the central nervous system, whereby depressive symptoms are reduced in relation to the reduction in inflammatory responses in the brain. These studies were carried out in 2014 in India and then in 2015 in China. In addition to the anti-inflammatory actions of its essential oil, it was also shown that Cumin has powerful pain management or analgesic properties.

Cuminaldehyde is one of the essential compounds in cumin thought to be useful in the management of cognitive decline and especially when considering Parkinson's disease. It was shown that the compound exhibited an inhibitory effect on alpha-synuclein fibrillation. This study from 2015 was a joint effort by scientists in Iran, Spain and Germany.

Another compound found in Cumin is safranal which is named after the plant Saffron as it was first isolated from this plant. As with Saffron (Crocus sativus), the presence of safranal in Cumin further gives support to the antidepressant use of the plant, and safranal is also recognised as having anti-inflammatory actions.

There are many other health claims associated with cumin, ranging from antibacterial to therapy for cancer management. However, two claims are of particular interest here. Research has shown that Cumin's essential oil significantly improves bowel function and reduces discomfort associated with Irritable Bowel Syndrome. As a result, the user of the essential oil for depression should be aware that their bowel function will change as well, fortunately for the better.

The other claim supported by clinical trials is the fact that its essential oil has also been shown to help in the reduction of weight and therefore the management of obesity. A study from 2014 in Iran showed that the essential oil reduced cholesterol, LDL and triglycerides while also decreasing the BMI for significantly overweight women. 88 obese women were involved in the trial and those women taking 3 grams of Cumin powder in yoghurt every day had similar weight loss when compared to the standard weight loss drug known as orlistat. The trial was conducted over 3 months, and no changes were made to either exercise regimes or diet during the period of the trial.

[1] M. East et al., "Cumin (/ ˈ k ʌ m ɪ n/, [2][3] / ˈ kju : m ɪ n/, [2][3] or."
[2] K. Srinivasan, "Cumin (Cuminum cyminum) and black cumin (Nigella sativa) seeds: Traditional uses, chemical constituents, and nutraceutical effects," Food Qual. Saf., vol. 2, no. 1, pp. 1–16, 2018.
[3] B. Muszyńska, M. Łojewski, J. Rojowski, W. Opoka, and K. Sułkowska-Ziaja, "Natural products of relevance in the prevention and supportive treatment of depression," Psychiatr. Pol., vol. 49, no. 3, pp. 435–453, 2015.
[4] A. E. Al-snafi, "The pharmacological activities of Cuminum cyminum -A review The pharmacological activities of Cuminum cyminum - A review Prof Dr Ali Esmail Al-Snafi," IOSR J. Pharm., vol. 6, no. 2, pp. 46–65, 2017.
[5] M. E. Ebada, "Cuminaldehyde: A Potential Drug Candidate," J. Pharmacol. Clin. Res., vol. 2, no. 2, 2017.

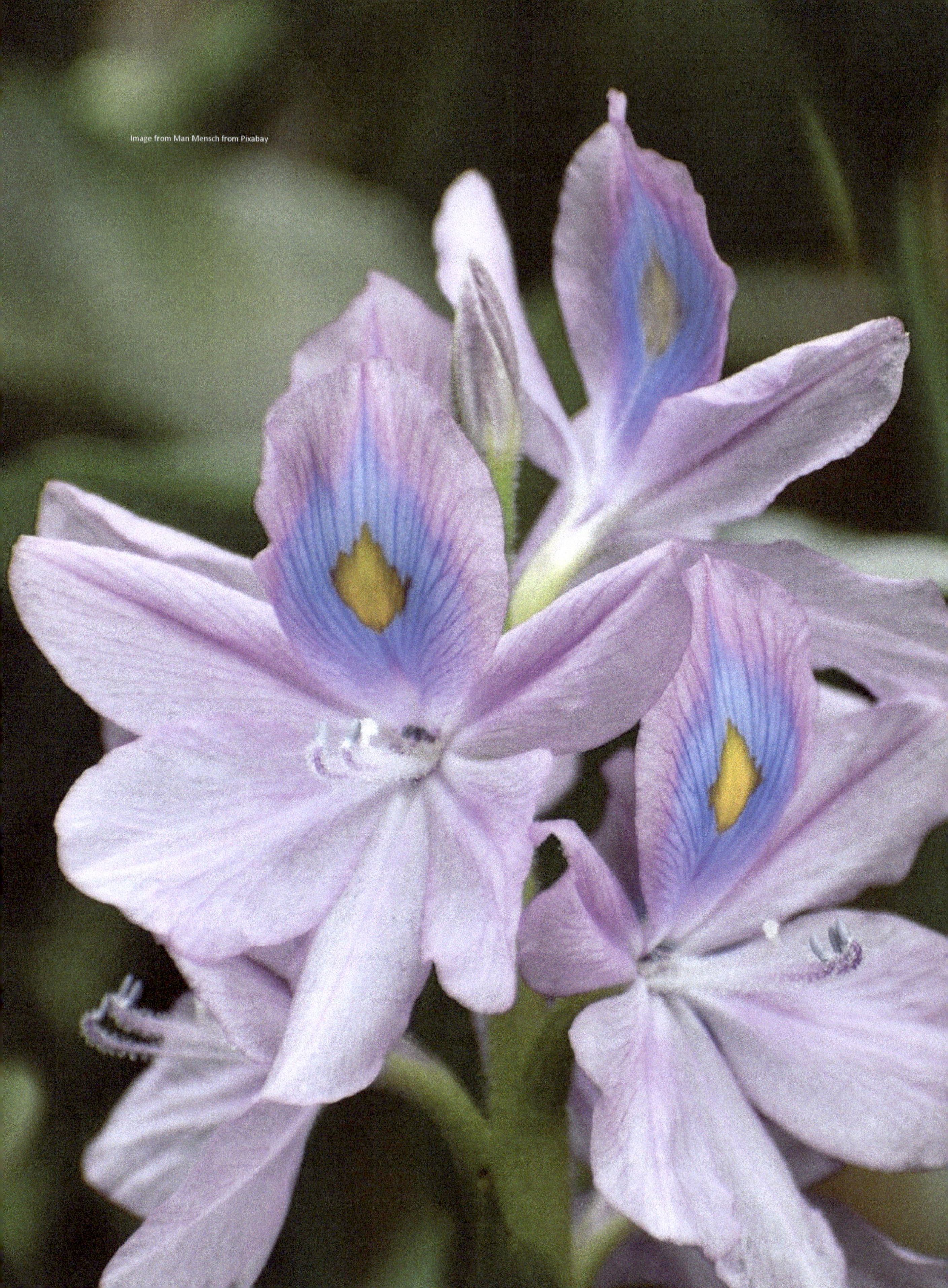

Image from Man Mensch from Pixabay

Common Water Hyacinth - Eichhornia crassipes

This is one of those stories that colour our world, the story of the Hippo and the South American flower.

Water Hyacinth has become one of the most invasive plants in the world. Originating from South America, specifically the Amazon basin, it has been transplanted to most countries around the world due to its ability to grow on water and its appealing flower. Today, it forms choking rafts on lakes, canals and waterways disrupting the native flora and fauna. It is known as one of the fastest growing plants in the world and is registered on many nation's invasive species lists. As a freshwater plant it is salt intolerant and in over 15% salt level of water it will die back. However, this was considered exorbitantly expensive in the application. As a result, in Louisiana in 1810, the American Hippo Bill (HR23621) was put forward by Congressman Robert Broussard allowing the African Hippopotamus to be imported and released into the waterways of Southern USA to eat the out of control plant. The bill failed by one vote.

The entire plant is edible, and in Vietnam, Taiwan and Indonesia the water hyacinth has been incorporated into diets. Other uses of the plant can be rope, furniture and baskets.

In 2015, researchers from Andhra Pradesh in India sought to test the antidepressant actions of the leaves and roots from the plant. They used the standard drug imipramine as a comparative control. In their testing, the test animals displayed a significant reduction in depressive symptomatology, and the findings from this paper endorsed the use of the plant for depression.

A more far reaching and extensive research paper was finalised in 2015 by researchers from Hyderabad, India, that sought to understand the neuroprotective, anxiolytic, antidepressant and anticonvulsant effects of both Eichhornia crassipes and Nymphaea Nelumbo (Lotus) compared to several standard pharmaceutical medicines. As a result, this research showed a significant support for the use of each plant and even more so when they were combined. It was shown that Eichhornia crassipes outperformed Lotus and both were comparable to diazepam, aspirin, ibuprofen, risperidone (antipsychotic), phenytoin (antiseizure) and chlorpromazine (antipsychotic). The findings showed that both plants resulted in positive results in the protection of brain neurons, a reduction in anxiety and depression, as well as mild pain relief and reduction in psychosis. Therefore, the Eichhornia crassipes is potentially a very useful source of medication for central nervous system disorders. In both of these research papers, the toxic levels of Water Hyacinth were researched, and the plant was found to be non-toxic, making it extremely safe to use, and eat.

Another useful aspect of Eichhornia crassipes is the antifungal properties of the plant. In a paper from the National Research Centre, Cairo, Egypt (2016), it was shown that leaf extract was highly effective in the control of various pathogenic fungal species.

[1] P. K. Uppala, K. Atchuta Kumar, S. K. Patro, and B. Murali Krishna, "Experimental evaluation of antidepressant activity of aqueous and chloroform leaf and shoot extracts of eicchornia crassipes linn in mice," Asian J. Pharm. Clin. Res., vol. 8, no. 5, pp. 241–244, 2015.

[2] M. Farheen and S. A. R. O. Hussaini, "Phytochemical Evaluation and Pharmacological Screening of Ethanolic Leaf Extracts of Eichhornia Crassipes and Nelumbo Nucifera for Neuropharmacological Activity in Psychoneurosis," vol. 4, no. 12, pp. 874–904, 2015.

[3] U. States, "Eichhornia crassipes," EPPO Bull., vol. 39, no. 3, pp. 460–464, 2009.

[4] Z. Rabiei and S. Rabie, "A review on antidepressant effect of medicinal plants," Bangladesh J. Pharmacol., vol. 12, no. 1, pp. 1–11, 2017.

Sportswear for depression

"You are gonna be happy, said Life, but first, I'll make you strong"

Anonymous

One of the most useless pieces of advice given to someone with depression comes from that well-meaning person who just wants to show you that they have absolutely no idea of what you are going through when they say, "It's a beautiful day! Common get outside. Go for a run. Get some exercise. It will make you feel better!" Even though they are right, they still remain a well-meaning idiot.

How could they know that depression waits out in that beautiful sunshine? It waits with one hundred-pound metaphorical bags. Ready to drop them on your shoulders as soon as you have those unused running shoes on. Depression is prancing beside you while you get the courage to simply jog faster than a walk, whispering in your ear, "You look ridiculous!" Depression is the personal anti-trainer. But! Depression is only on one channel, and you have the right to change channels. It's not easy, but the trick is taking your time.

One company stumbled into the sportswear market with what later became the anthem for the sports depressed. In 1987, Nike reluctantly adopted the slogan "Just Do It!" that was coined by Dan Weiden of the advertising firm Weiden+Kennedy. The story goes that Dan while preparing for the presentation to the Nike team the next day, thought he needed a tagline to tie the disparate pieces of the proposed campaign together. After some thought, Dan drew inspiration from a very unlikely source and presented it to the room during the presentation. The story further states that no one really liked the term but accepted that they should try it for one season and then dump it. Twenty years later and more, the tagline is still in use. As it so happens, Dan took it from the last words of the convicted killer, Gary Gilmore, who famously said when facing the firing squad in Ohio 1977 shrugged his shoulders and simply stated "Let's do it!"

"Just Do It!" is the best and most elegantly simple argument a depressive sufferer has. Stop thinking. Stop procrastinating. Stop feeling sorry for yourself and just do it. Nike had become the sportswear maker for the depressed, without actually knowing it. The trick is to stop thinking and just exercise.

Exercise has been shown to have dramatic effects on the body across the board. Physically, emotionally, and intellectually. There have been dozens of research papers written on the impact of exercise and reduction in depression in the young as well as the elderly. One report from Brazil in 2016 reviewed a range of other research papers focusing on the effects of exercise on the elderly (65+ years) and concluded that both aerobic and strength training had significant results in reducing depressive episodes. The report went even further to suggest that exercise may replace the need for antidepressant drugs in this age group. Statistically, exercise is shown to be a powerful tool for controlling depression. It has also been found that older people who did not exercise had an 83% higher chance of developing depression. Other studies have displayed the benefits of exercise in all age groups. Another research study found children who had high levels of physical activity had 38% less risk of developing depression. And yet, another study from Norway found that men and women who exercised regularly respectively had a 37% and 31% reduction in depressive symptoms. In all the studies, it was found that different cultures and ethnic backgrounds all showed the same benefits from regular physical activity.

With all this interest in why exercise had such a profound effect in improving depression, it was thought that it was due to the body releasing endorphins. However, this has been discounted somewhat over the years as more and more physical changes have been witnessed as a result of exercise. Of these changes in the body, the improvement of cognitive function has been substantiated repeatedly, and it has been shown that exercise actually increases certain areas of the brain, most specifically the outer layer of the cerebrum. A lowering of inflammation in the body is also one of the benefits of exercise. The increase in oxygen in the body due to cardio exercise is also cited as a possible reason for the reduction in depressive symptoms. All in all, the benefits of both cardiovascular exercise and resistance exercise have been substantiated universally, yet the most straightforward reason may merely be the improvement of self-image as people lose weight and take better care of themselves.

Sadly, depression manifests itself as low motivation, lethargy, lack of interest and general fatigue which all make it incredibly hard for a sufferer to get off the couch or out of bed and actually start an exercise regime and keep to it. Many people have developed tricks or hacks to jump-start their own recovery from depression and in some cases have made quite a bit of money and fame by writing books about them, conducting classes or giving lectures. One of these is the '5-second rule' developed by Mel Robbins, where she recommends counting down from 5 to 1 immediately after which a decision to act must be made. Another simple, yet powerful technique was developed by Wim Hof who strongly recommends a deep breathing regime in order to improve not only depression but all aspects of your body and mind. Further, another is the WTF technique that promises that all one has to do is to get ready to exercise as the bare minimum a person has to do each day. This technique relies upon a person getting dressed to exercise and standing outside their door as a bare minimum, and if they still don't feel like going for that run or going to the gym then that's alright, at least they got ready for it. This technique relies on the simple fact that once you are in your gym or running gear and outside your door, you will then hit the WTF button and go for that run anyway and take your dog with you. The trick is to find the technique that works for you.

The findings in research and studies on the effects of exercise, as to how much and for how long you should exercise, have also been studied. The results confirm that a person should exercise at least three times per week and the optimum number of times is five times. Each session should be for no less than forty-five minutes and the optimum of sixty minutes, for ten weeks. In reality, a person should continue exercising for years and not worry about seeing results at any time, because this expectation of quick results is prone to demoralise or depress a person when the results don't manifest as quickly as wanted.

[1] P. C. Dinas, Y. Koutedakis, and A. D. Flouris, 'Effects of exercise and physical activity on depression,' Ir. J. Med. Sci., vol. 180, no. 2, pp. 319–325, 2011.

[2] F. B. Schuch et al., 'Exercise for depression in older adults: A meta-analysis of randomized controlled trials adjusting for publication bias,' Rev. Bras. Psiquiatr., vol. 38, no. 3, pp. 247–254, 2016.

[3] M. B. Murri et al., 'Physical exercise in major depression: Reducing the mortality gap while improving clinical outcomes,' Front. Psychiatry, vol. 9, no. January, pp. 1–10, 2019.

[4] F. B. Schuch, B. Stubbs, F. B. Schuch, and B. Stubbs, 'Physical Activity, Physical Fitness, and Depression,' Oxford Res. Encycl. Psychol., no. October, 2017.

[5] LAST, 'Foundations , Promises and Uncertainties of Personalized Medicine Address Correspondence to :,' Medicine (Baltimore)., pp. 15–21, 2007.

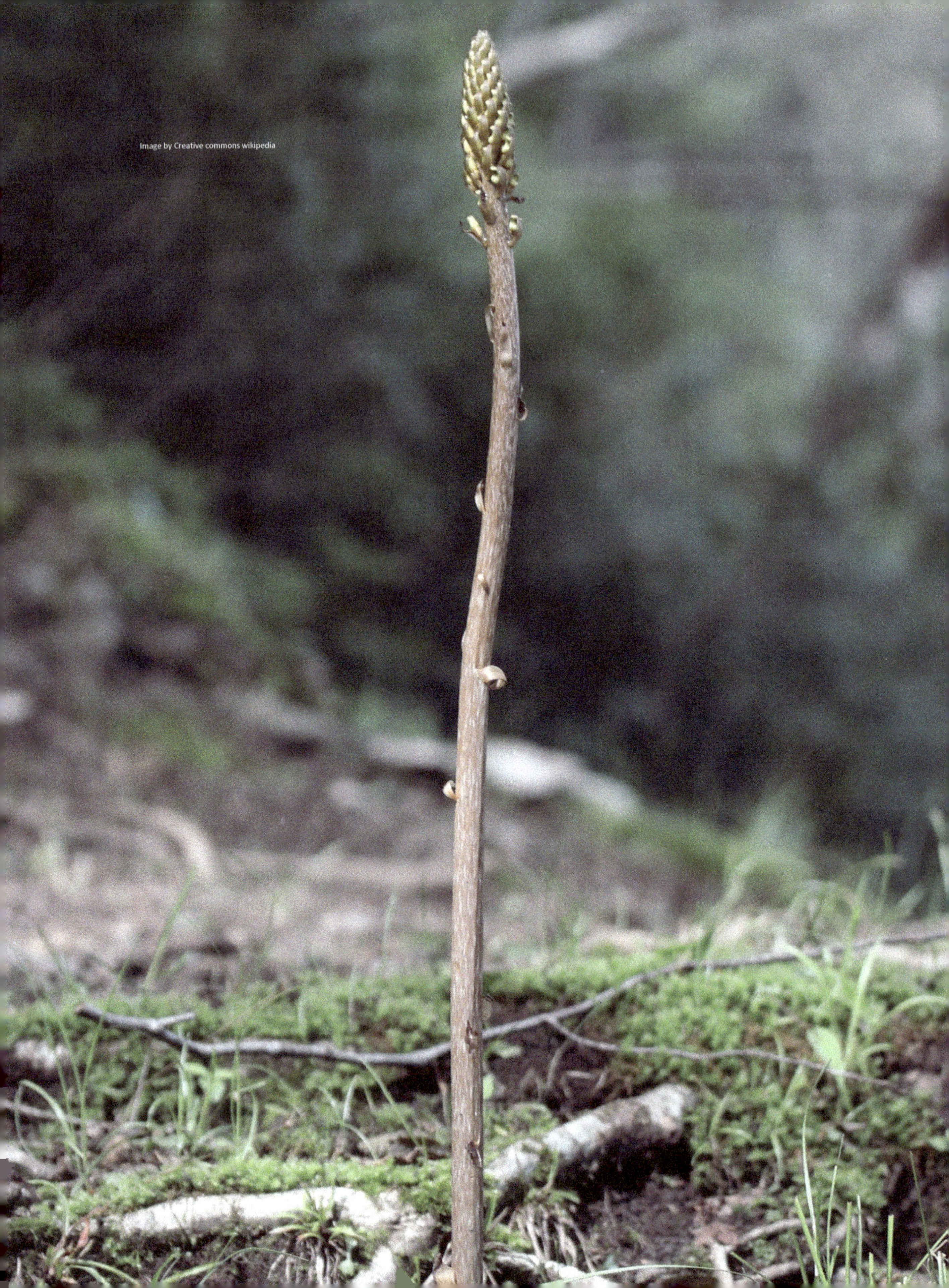
Image by Creative commons wikipedia

Tianma - Gastrodia elata

Gastrodia elata is a mainstay herb in the Chinese pharmacopoeia and has been used for centuries in the central and western regions of Asia. The herb is found from Nepal, Bhutan, India, Japan, China, Siberia, Taiwan and South Korea. Unfortunately, most of the supply of this plant comes from wild harvesting as it exists in symbiosis with the fungus Armillaria mellea which feeds on rotting timber. Gastrodia elata is a member of the Orchid family and is a saprophyte.

In Chinese herbal medicine it is believed that Gastrodia works via the liver channels, and is used to treat dizziness, epilepsy, paralysis, lethargy and generally prolongs life. The compounds found within the plant that are thought to be responsible for its medicinal actions are gastrodin, gastrol, gastrodigenin, vanillin and S-4- glutathione.

There has been a great deal of research into the actions and applications of Gastrodia over the years, and much of the work has endorsed its applications in medicine. Yet its significant effect on the central nervous system makes it unique.

A report published in the American Journal of Chinese Medicine from 2009 discussed the role of the plant in the management of depression. In this report a team of scientists from several universities in Taiwan combined their efforts and found that the simple water extract of the tuber from the plant was as effective as fluoxetine in the management of symptoms of depression.

Other clinical studies from the early 2000's supported claims that the water extract from the plant showed significant anti-inflammatory actions as well as anticonvulsant properties. These findings add further support to the benefits of using the herb for central nervous systems support. Allied with this is the reported mediation of free radicals and the resulting oxidation stress on the tissue.

It has been further shown that the use of the plant extract increases the dopamine levels in the brain. This monoamine dopamine is called the 'reward' neurotransmitter, but synthetically increased levels of it may result in addiction. Lowered levels of dopamine are also associated with depression as sufferers fail to see rewards from positive action. The extract apparently did not elevate the serotonin levels. However, an earlier study on anxiety management, achieved by the use of the water extract from the roots of the plant, showed the possible association with the serotonergic system in the reduction of anxiety in test animals. Here again we find the research compelling, however the underlying mechanisms of the plants are challenging to pinpoint.

The plant has been shown to have pain reduction abilities as well, which may endorse its classical use in the management of headaches.

Doses of between 500-1000 mg/kg body weight have been recommended of the water extract. This may be reduced should an ethanol or methanol extraction process be used.

[1] P. J. Chen, C. L. Hsieh, K. P. Su, Y. C. Hou, H. M. Chiang, and L. Y. Sheen, "Rhizomes of Gastrodia elata BL possess antidepressant-like effect via monoamine modulation in subchronic animal model," Am. J. Chin. Med., vol. 37, no. 6, pp. 1113–1124, 2009.

[2] P. J. Chen et al., "The antidepressant effect of Gastrodia elata Bl. on the forced-swimming test in rats," Am. J. Chin. Med., vol. 36, no. 1, pp. 95–106, 2008.

[3] "Gastrodia Elata Bl on Phencyclidine-Induced Schizophrenia-Like Psychosis.".

[4] "Antidepressant effects of Gastrodia elata Bl."

[5] "Anxiolytic-Like Effects of Gastrodia elata."

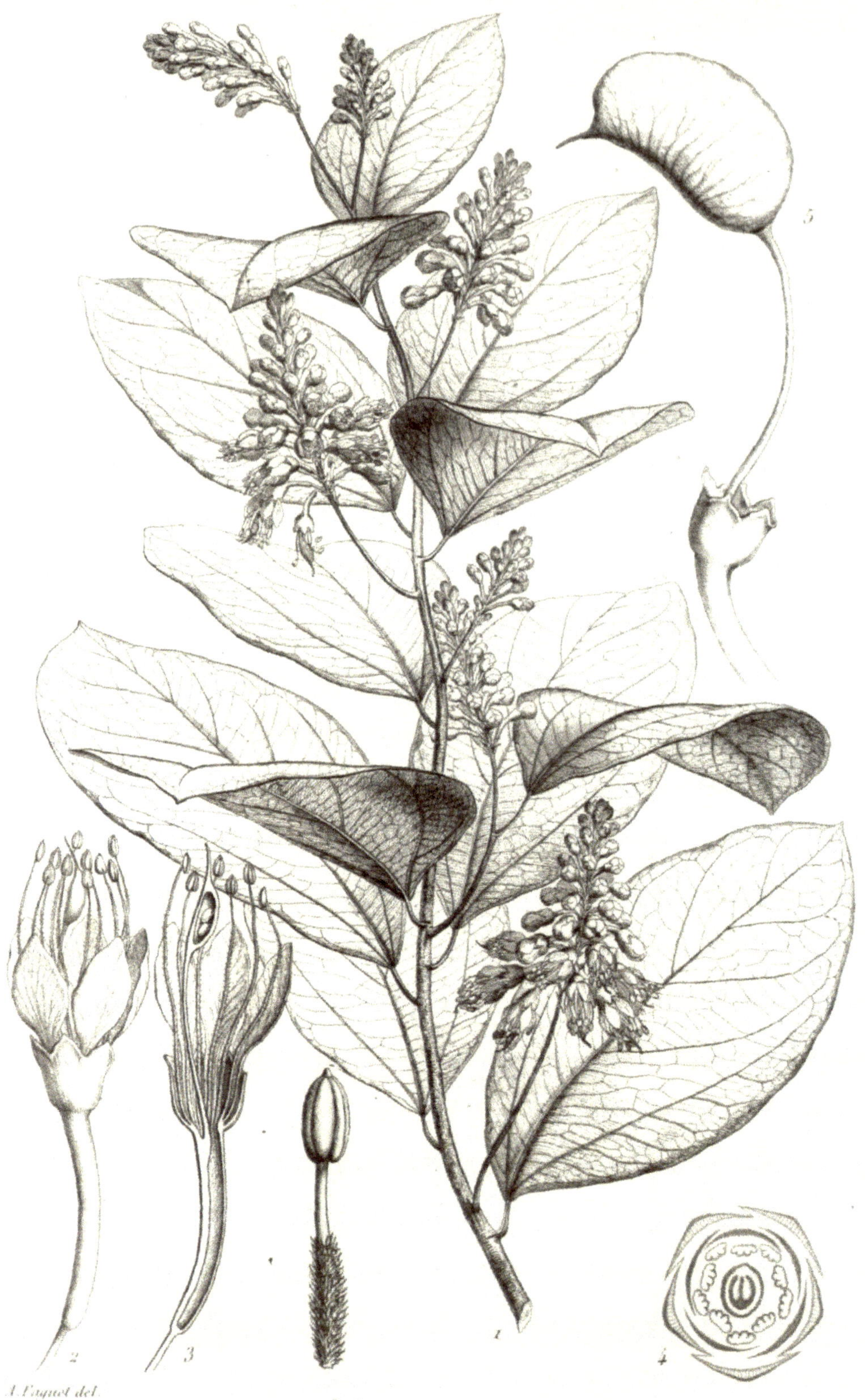

1. Griffonia simplicifolia 2_5. G. physocarpa

Kayja / Atootoo - Griffonia simplicifolia

Griffonia is a climbing shrub found on the west coast of Africa and primarily in Ghana, Ivory Coast, Togo, Liberia and Gabon. It has been used for centuries by its local people for a range of health applications, however more recently, it has gained prominence as an antidepressant and anti-anxiety medication.

The plant has large glabrous seed pods that appear to be far too large for the small seeds contained within them. It is the seed of the plant that is harvested for commercial purposes, and a paper (2010) described how the seeds are primarily gathered from the wild with little or no commercial plantings. As a result, there are concerns that the plant is being overharvested and may not have a sustainable future. The majority of the seeds harvested are destined for the European or US markets where they are refined into a concentrated form and sold under various trade names specifically for mood enhancement.

Research has found that the seeds are a rich source of 5-hydroxitryptophan (5-HTP) which is the main building block in the body for the synthesis of serotonin, one of the primary neurotransmitters associated with mental health and well-being. It is interesting to note that there is a widespread use of 5-HTP by the users of MDMA, commonly known as ecstasy, a drug taken by people for a feeling of euphoria and happiness. People who consume MDMA do so before a dance or rave party. Not surprisingly, they suffer from what is known as the post-MDMA dysphoria afterwards as Isaac Newton claimed, "For each action there is a equal and opposite reaction!"

Chinese research from 2013 found new unique compounds in Griffonia which they named griffonine and which are in the beta-carboline family of alkaloids. Members of this group have been associated with psychoactive properties and may positively influence the pineal gland's sleep-wake cycle. Traditionally the seed extract has been used to moderate insomnia.

Griffonia simplicifolia seed extract has also been used to balance weight levels in both obese and anorexic people, as it is thought that the 5-HTP regulates the feelings of appetite in both. In one research study a dosage of between 25-100 mg of Griffonia resulted in an average reduction in food intake by test animals by 33%. So, if you are one of the depressed people who find solace in food, Griffonia might be the more suitable antidepressant medication that you are looking for.

As an anti-anxiety medication Griffonia has also been compared to the standard drug diazepam, and whilst the plant extract did show significant anti-anxiety effects, it was not as effective as diazepam.

Research of 2019 into the possible toxicity of Griffonia use showed that doses up to 5000 mg/kg were considered non-toxic, and as a result the use of the herb is considered safe.

Various plants synthesise either 5-HTP or serotonin as a defence against insects.

[1] P. S. Kumar, T. Praveen, and B. Jitendra, "A review on Griffonia simplicifollia - an ideal herbal anti-depressant," Int. J. Pharm. Life Sci., vol. 1, no. 3, pp. 174–181, 2010.

[2] R. A. Nyarko, C. Larbie, A. K. Anning, and P. Kweku Baidoo, "Phytochemical Constituents, Antioxidant Activity and Toxicity Assessment of Hydroethanolic Leaf Extract of Griffonia Simplicifolia," Int. J. Phytopharm. Res. Artic., vol. 10, no. 1, pp. 6–18, 2019.

[3] D. Giurleo, "©2017 Daniel Giurleo All Rights Reserved," 2017.

[4] I. Vigliante, G. Mannino, and M. E. Maffei, "Chemical characterization and DNA fingerprinting of griffonia simplicifolia baill," Molecules, vol. 24, no. 6, 2019.

Diet

"I drank to drown my pain, but the damned pain learned how to swim..."

Frida Kahlo

We have been told that "We are what we eat". In the case of depression, the saying should be re-written to more precisely reflect the truth by stating "We feel what we eat", or perhaps 'Mood food'. The link between diet and depression is nowadays well and truly cast, yet, whilst not precisely clear, it is better understood.

The human body is comprised of a multitude of compounds or building blocks per se. Some of these compose the structure of the body, carbon, oxygen, hydrogen, nitrogen etc. They are known as the major elements that make up the bulk of the body at 96%. Others are known as the semi-major elements such as potassium, sodium etc. and account for 3-4% of our mass. The smallest of these are the trace elements and they make up only 0.02%. They however play a critical role as bioactive substances that regulate bodily function, especially when we consider mental or psychological performance.

Let's consider the bipolar medication lithium. A safe level of this metal in our bodies is .00006 to .00012 parts per litre, yet a minute rise in the level of lithium of .00004 parts per litre can be life-threatening. Therefore, we can use the example of lithium to highlight that even small deficiencies of trace elements can have profound impacts on our physical and mental health.

A poor diet can manifest depression due to a reduction of trace elements. When we are actually in a depressive state, the last thing we think about is eating a balanced and healthy diet. All we want is comfort food and treats, whether they are sugars, cigarettes, or alcohol. As such, our diets can lead us into depression and then keep us there unless we understand what is actually going on. Of course, there is a universal gap between knowing we should have a healthy diet and actually implementing one. The reality is probably more like, "Ahh ... fuck it, give me chocolate". That glass of wine that leads to another one, and then finally to going to bed without eating solid food is all too common. So, with such confessions, it is probably more useful to commence with over-the-counter supplements until such time as the interest and discipline of maintaining a healthy diet arises. Unravelling the puzzle of which elements are crucial for mood improvement, and what shifts are required to happiness, is the discussion here.

A complex compound is just that ... complex. The body requires building blocks to be available so that they can be built. If we consider serotonin for example, a key ingredient for this monoamine to be made in the body is the amino acid L-tryptophan. Another element is phenylalanine and it is essential for the formation of dopamine. Without these two, it would be guaranteed that a body would have low levels of each. Luckily, you can buy supplements of both these amino acids. Obviously, they are only two ingredients out of many that are essential for the making of an anti-depression salad. After a quick research, a few, if any, multivitamins on the market were found that were either a) specifically formulated for depression, and or b) contained sufficient ingredients within them to be optimal in effect. I could provide you with a list of vitamins and minerals and be done with it, however, it is suggested you know and comprehend them all, as like what Krishna Murti stated, "In the land of truth there are no paths". That one important key ingredient to defeating depression is knowledge. Knowledge so that you can find your path out of the ennui of despair. You should not simply follow someone else's footsteps. They did not start where you began.

We can dispense with simplicity here. There are far too many fads and expert recommendations. Opinions abound not just from experts but also from backyard gurus spruiking the latest and greatest cure or remedy. Let's just settle down comfortably on the couch of science and cushions of facts, so that in the end we will know that there is no doubt about what we should and shouldn't eat.

Within our bodies, our chemistry can create enzymes and other compounds from simple chemical components that we have consumed via eating, drinking, and even breathing. However, in some cases this is not possible, and as a result we need essential ingredients, as is the case with the essential amino acids. There are nine essential amino acids, two of which are crucial for the production of serotonin and dopamine. Again, in short, there are hormones or neurotransmitters involved in promoting a happy mood and positive feelings, and you might know serotonin as the happiness hormone, dopamine as the feel-good hormone, and a third, oxytocin is also known as the cuddle hormone.

L-Tryptophan is not only essential for the synthesis of serotonin but also for melatonin, another neurotransmitter necessary for healthy sleep patterns. Niacin, also known as vitamin B3, is also derived from tryptophan, and this vitamin is critical for the energy transfer reactions in the metabolism of glucose, fat and alcohol. As a result, a diet low in this amino acid will have a dramatic impact on mood, sleep, and energy. The recommended daily intake of L-tryptophan is between 27 mg and 476 mg. Foods that are high in L-tryptophan are turkey breast, chicken breast, milk, tinned tuna, and oats etc. A piece of good news here is the understanding that chocolate is also listed as a food high in this essential ingredient. Sadly, before you reach for that large block of sugary pleasure, the levels of L-tryptophan in chocolate are not high enough for you to get your daily intake without also ending up the size of a whale. At any rate, you can feel a little bit better when you indulge your chocolate craving. As we can see, this amino acid is critical for the serotonin levels in the body. If you are already taking a serotonin re-uptake inhibiting drug or (SSRI's), then care should be taken as serotonin levels may exceed a healthy level and Serotonin Syndrome may result.

Phenylalanine is another essential amino acid that our bodies cannot make. Yet, this time this amino acid is required for the synthesis of dopamine, the pleasure hormone, as well as adrenaline and norepinephrine, and therefore it makes this amino acid as crucial as tryptophan if not possibly more crucial. Only by increasing their levels, these two will have a significant effect on the function of your neurotransmitters, and as a result a decrease in depressive symptoms. Phenylalanine is required for the synthesis of another amino acid tyrosine which in turn is used to synthesize dopamine, adrenaline, and norepinephrine. Phenylalanine is found in eggs, soybeans, chicken, fish, certain nuts and strangely in high levels in the artificial sweetener aspartame.

Choline is not an essential nutrient. Whilst the body can produce it, the levels produced are not sufficient for good health. Sometimes choline is called vitamin B4, yet this is incorrect, as it is not considered to be part of the B group. Choline is vital in the production of the neurotransmitter acetylcholine as well as aiding the body in the production of cell membranes and plasma lipoproteins. Acetylcholine is of the same importance as the other monoamines serotonin, dopamine and norepinephrine.

Thiamine – vitamin B1 adds to the suite of B vitamins and their role in emotional and physical health. Thiamine deficiency is most associated with the medical condition known as beriberi which is a condition where the nerves of the body become inflamed, and this may result in eventual heart failure. Immediately we see the link with depression due to the inflammation of the nervous system. As a result, this vitamin is definitely on our list of must-haves. Thiamine supplementation has shown improved sleep patterns.

Niacin – vitamin B3, while its positive influence on depression has long been accepted, the reason why is still unclear. Regardless, niacin supplementation has shown good results in the treatment of depression as far back as the 1950s. Niacin overdose may manifest as skin flushing, diarrhoea, rapid heartbeat, gout, and vomiting.

Pantothenic acid – vitamin B5 is a critical ingredient in the formation or development of neurotransmitters. Sources of this vitamin are chicken, beef, pork, eggs, vegetables of the cabbage family such as broccoli and kale, mushrooms, and beans.

Pyridoxine - vitamin B6 acts similarly to vitamin B5 in that it is an ingredient in the biosynthesis of neurotransmitters. Sources for this vitamin are similar to pantothenic acid with the addition of cereals such as wheat, oats, rice, and others. Pyridoxine excess may be felt in the following manner: light sensitivity, numbness, and loss of control of muscles.

Biotin – vitamin B7, like the other B vitamins it has a diverse role in the human body. Findings have shown that a deficiency of Biotin is associated with depression, lethargy, hallucinations and seizures. It is a rare condition to have if you eat a healthy diet. The converse is true if you eat too many processed foods and too many egg whites because this inhibits the absorption of vitamin B7. The irony here is that egg white is a good source of biotin but only when they are cooked. In a study from 2019 it was found that during pregnancy the biotin levels in women decreased significantly as this vitamin is essential in the development of the fetus. This may be a contributing factor to postpartum depression. Other causes of biotin deficiency are smoking, liver disease, alcohol abuse, and ketogenic diets (low carbohydrate and high-fat diets). Skin rashes may appear if you are taking too much biotin.

Folate – vitamin B9 is thought to interact and support the serotonergic and noradrenergic systems, and as such it has long been thought to alleviate depressive symptoms. It is believed that one-third of patients who suffer from depression are folate deficient. Also notable is the role folate plays in foetal development. The primary source of folate is green leafy vegetables, fruits, and legumes. The recommended daily allowance of folate is thought to be 400 micrograms per day.

Cobalamin – vitamin B12 has a broad range of actions in the body. From being involved with cellular metabolism of carbohydrates, proteins, and fats to nerve function and health. Cobalamin has long been associated with mood disorders, especially for major depression that does not respond to the standard antidepressants. It has been discussed in a research paper from 2013 that a significant proportion of patients respond positively to B12 supplementation in the treatment of major depression. For those who have a deficiency with this vitamin, it is recommended to start with a dose of 300 mcg once per day and then drop to a maintenance dose of between 100-200 mcg per day. Less than 10% of those studied have adverse reactions to high levels of this vitamin and reactions such as joint pain, headaches, and dizziness. Skin lesions, thirst, increased urination, blurry vision, diarrhoea and nausea may be experienced.

Magnesium plays a role in over 300 enzymatic reactions. It is essential for nerve impulse and transmission in the brain and central nervous system. Magnesium is also vital in the metabolism of food with particular emphasis on the synthesis of fatty acids, (which are also crucial in the treatment of depression) and proteins. The human body contains approximately 25 grams of magnesium, most of which is stored in the bones (50-60%). A daily dose of around 350 mg of magnesium is thought to be sufficient. Too much magnesium may result in thirst, cardiac arrhythmia, diarrhoea, weakness, difficulty in breathing and coma.

Zinc is another vital micronutrient that has been shown to be effective in the treatment of depression, primarily where supplementation occurs with other pharmaceutical regimes. Similar to magnesium, it is thought that zinc is involved in over 300 enzymatic processes. Zinc is called a transition metal as it is required for gene expression, hormonal storage, tissue repair, DNA replication, protein synthesis and cellular signalling. Zinc is a molecule found in high levels throughout the central nervous system. A therapeutic dose is considered to be 200 mg per day for a first dose and then a reference dose of 3-11 mg per day after that. Yet, zinc may be more critical and effective in treating depression in women than men as it has been found a more vital link between zinc deficiency within women. Too much may result in nausea, stomach pain, diarrhoea, flu-like symptoms, increased bad cholesterol, copper and iron deficiency, and frequent infections.

Selenium is used to improve mood and depressive symptoms in daily doses of around 100 micrograms per day, however, a more conservative daily dose of 55 micrograms per day is recommended. Selenium is taken up by plants, yet this also depends on the selenium levels in the soil in which the plants grow. Some regions of the world have extremely low levels, and various health conditions associated with low selenium levels are evident in them. Selenium aids in the production of sperm, support of the immune system and cardiac health. More research has shown a clear link between selenium levels and mood. The thyroid gland has the highest levels of selenium in the body, and as such it is thought to be critical in the synthesis of thyroid hormones. There are contradicting findings from research as it was shown that selenium supplements improved the efficacy of fluoxetine, a standard antidepressant drug, yet other research has argued the opposite and claims selenium reduces the effectiveness of this drug. Care should be used in the prescribing of selenium as high doses can be toxic and cause nail discolouration/loss, hair loss, foul breath, fatigue, and irritability.

Manganese also aids the thyroid and is vital in the synthesis of the thyroid hormone thyroxine. It is also essential for nerve impulse transfer in the brain and central nervous system. As such, it can improve cognitive function and reduce anxiety. Care should be taken however as manganese is easy to overdose on. Symptoms of overdose may be tremors, loss of appetite, and reproductive issues. A daily intake of 2 mg per day is recommended. Too much manganese may have side effects such as irritability, aggressiveness, hallucinations, tremors and facial muscle spasms. Manganese is an abundant metal here on earth, and we can absorb it via air, water, and food. As such, probably, you are already receiving enough of this mineral.

Iron, its deficiency causes anaemia, a reduction in healthy red blood cells and the resulting dangerous reduction of oxygen to the cells of the body. The symptoms of anaemia are lethargy, weakness and low motivation, and closely resemble depression. However, iron is also required for the processing of L-tryptophan and tyrosine. A deficiency of this mineral will exacerbate depression. Food high in iron are dark leafy vegetables, beans, lentils, tofu, potato and cashew nuts. A therapeutic dose of iron is thought to be 325 mg of ferrous sulphate or ferrous gluconate per day. Too much iron may result in fatigue, skin colour changes, liver damage, black stool, joint pain, abdominal pain, and irregular heart rhythm. Iron and zinc impede each other. As a result, it is a bad idea to take them at the same time.

Chromium has a mixed history with researchers when it comes to its efficacy in the treatment of depression. Some papers endorse its use in the treatment of depression enthusiastically, yet others remain doubtful. Regardless, for our purposes we will accept the bulk view that chromium is highly effective in reducing the burden of depression. A recent research document on the effectiveness of chromium leaves no doubt in this regard. A dose of 600 micrograms per day was the regime used in the research paper quoted here. Chromium overdose may exhibit the following symptoms, cramps, vertigo, nausea, vomiting, and gastric ulcers.

Iodine is vital for good thyroid function as it is required for the synthesis of growth-regulating thyroid hormones, thyroxine and triiodothyronine. Deficiency in iodine levels in the body may be felt as fatigue, mental slowing, depression, weight gain and low body temperature. Food high in this element is seafood (such as fish and shellfish), seaweeds, eggs, and dairy products. The recommended daily intake of iodine for adults is thought to be 150 micrograms per day. Iodine toxicity manifests with the following symptoms: burning of the mouth, throat and stomach, fever, nausea, diarrhoea, and weak pulse.

Omega-3 fatty acids cannot be made by the body and therefore must be sourced through the food we eat. As such omega-3 fatty acids are considered to be essential in much the same way as the two amino acids tryptophan and phenylalanine. Seafood, flaxseed, and hemp oil are the highest sources of omega-3 fatty acids. Scientific research has shown a clear link between lower levels of omega-3 and depression. Our modern diets are becoming omega-3 deficient as we move to more intensive farming of livestock and seafood. As a result, we are having an imbalance between omega-3 and omega-6 fatty acids, where omega-3 is anti-inflammatory, and omega-6 stimulates inflammation. A recommended daily dose of omega-3 is between 1-2 grams per day. Cholesterol-lowering drugs named statins interfere with omega-3 levels in the body, and their use may bring on depressive episodes.

Vitamin D – more precisely known as cholecalciferol is a bit of a controversial compound. For starters, it is not really considered either a vitamin or a mineral but rather a prohormone or a substance that the human body converts into a true hormone. In the case of vitamin D, the majority of this compound is produced in the skin as cholecalciferol which is then further processed in the liver into calcifediol. Finally, the kidneys turn this into calcitriol which is the active hormone. The remaining 10% found in the body we get from our food, such as dairy and fatty fish. Once again, there are counterclaims as to the efficacy of vitamin D in depression therapy. One such paper casts doubt as to the effectiveness of treating non-clinical depression with this compound. Yet, in the same article, the researchers agree that there is evidence that it does indeed have a positive effect on clinical depression. This paper is confusing in its own right, making it more difficult for people like you and I to unravel claims and counterclaims. Albeit vitamin D is essential in the absorption of magnesium as well as calcium and in so doing must therefore have a positive effect. Other research has shown vitamin D highly beneficial in the treatment of fatigue and chronic fatigue syndrome. This factor alone makes it of interest to the depressed person who is finding it hard to get motivated. Other research has shown that vitamin D has a positive supporting role for the functioning of serotonin, dopamine, norepinephrine and other monoamines. Too much vitamin D may cause hypercalcaemia or dangerously high levels of calcium in the body that may cause other health complications.

With the above list of amino acids, vitamins and minerals, a supplementary regime becomes clearer and may be used in conjunction with other therapeutic medicines. However, some confusion may arise when considering a 'therapeutic dose' compared to the 'recommended dietary allowance'

(RDA). The latter is commonly found printed on the labels of supplements purchased at a retail outlet or chemist. The RDA is defined as 'the levels of intake of essential nutrients that, based on scientific knowledge, are judged by the Food and Nutrition Board to be adequate to meet the known nutrient needs of practically all healthy persons.' Yet, we assume that a depressed person is 1 not healthy and 2 lacking in one or more of the listed supplements above. A therapeutic dose is therefore required to correct the imbalance, such a dose is defined as follows, 'The quantity of any substance to effect the cure of a disease or to correct the manifestation of a deficiency of a particular factor in the diet'.

If required, a simple blood test may be done to check on the levels of these vitamins and minerals or merely a regime of additional supplements for a period of not less than 14 days at the end of which a positive development in mood would indicate a continuation of the supplements themselves. The table below outlines the therapeutic dose and RDA and the upper safe dose.

It is essential to understand a dramatic yet beautiful law, of not merely medicine but also a 'law of life'. It can be stated as "The therapy taken in the correct dose may act like a medicine and result in a cure, however, should excessive amounts of the same medicine be taken, the medicine will transform into poison and result in the exact opposite". Therefore, any substance, and in this case vitamins and minerals, may cause harm if taken in excessive doses. Lithium is a clear example. Likewise, magnesium, manganese, chromium, selenium and others should be taken in the correct amount only.

Supplement	**Recommended Dietary Allowance (RDA)**	**Therapeutic Dose**	**Upper Safe Limit (USL)**
Tryptophan	5 mg/kg	278 mg	476 mg[3]
Phenylalanine	33 mg	20 mg	40 mg[14]
Choline	550 mg	-	3,500 mg
Biotin	30 micrograms	2.5 mg	15 mg[15]
Cobalamin	2.4 micrograms	25 micrograms	2000 micrograms
Folate	400 micrograms	400 micrograms	800 micrograms[16]
Niacin	16 mg	1000 mg	1000 mg[17]
Pantothenic acid	5 mg	200 mg	1000 mg[18]
Pyridoxine	1.3 mg	100 mg	500 mg[19]
Thiamine	1.2 mg	15 mg	50 mg[20]
Magnesium	310 gm (F) - 400 gm (M)	310 gm (F) – 400 gm (M)	310 gm(F) – 400 gm (M)[21]
Zinc	8 mg (F) - 11 gm (M)	50 mg	600 mg[22]
Selenium	55 micrograms	150 micrograms	1 0 micrograms[23]
Manganese	1.8 mg (F) - 2.8 gm (M)	10 mg	25 mg/kgpd
Iron	12 mg (F) - 18 mg (M)	50 mg	120 mg
Chromium	25 mcg (F)-35 mcg (M)	50 micrograms	1000 micrograms
Iodine	150 micrograms	250 micrograms	1000 micrograms
Omega-3 fatty acid	1.1 gm (F) - 1.6 gm (M)	2.5 gms	5000 mg
Vitamin D	600-800 IU per day	100,000 IU	-

(F) = female (M) = male

[1] O. Wada, 'What are Trace Elements ? — Their deficiency and excess states,' Jpn Med Assoc J, vol. 47, no. 5, p. 351, 2004.
[2] T. Sathyanarayana Rao, M. Asha, B. Ramesh, and K. Jagannatha Rao, 'Understanding nutrition, depression and mental illnesses,' Indian J. Psychiatry, vol. 50, no. 2, p. 77, 2008.
[3] D. M. Richard, M. A. Dawes, C. W. Mathias, A. Acheson, N. Hill-Kapturczak, and D. M. Dougherty, 'L-tryptophan: Basic metabolic functions, behavioural research and therapeutic indications,' Int. J. Tryptophan Res., vol. 2, no. 1, pp. 45–60, 2009.
[4] SMO, 'Biotin deficiency,' J. Nutr. Educ., vol. 13, no. 3, p. 96, 1981.
[5] E. U. Syed, M. Wasay, and S. Awan, 'Vitamin B12 Supplementation in Treating Major Depressive Disorder: A Randomized Controlled Trial,' Open Neurol. J., vol. 7, no. 1, pp. 44–48, 2013.
[6] E. H. Reynolds, 'Folic acid, ageing, depression, and dementia,' vol. 324, no. June 2002.
[7] K. Slawinska, G. Bielecka, K. Iwaniak, S. Wosko, and E. Poleszak, 'Selenium and manganese in depression – Preclinical and clinical studies,' Curr. Issues Pharm. Med. Sci., vol. 30, no. 3, pp. 151–155, 2017.
[8] S. M. Aburawi and S. A. Baayo, 'Behavior Effect of Fluoxetine in Presence of Selenium Using Albino Mice,' Int. J. Pharmacol. Phytochem. Ethnomedicine, vol. 7, pp. 1–8, 2017.
[9] S. Hidese, K. Saito, S. Asano, and H. Kunugi, 'Association between iron-deficiency anaemia and depression: A web-based Japanese investigation,' Psychiatry Clin. Neurosci., vol. 72, no. 7, pp. 513–521, 2018.
[10] M. N. McLeod and R. N. Golden, 'Chromium treatment of depression,' Int. J. Neuropsychopharmacol., vol. 3, no. 4, pp. 311–314, 2000.
[11] J. R. T. Davidson, K. Abraham, K. M. Connor, and M. N. McLeod, 'Effectiveness of chromium in atypical depression: A placebo-controlled trial,' Biol. Psychiatry, vol. 53, no. 3, pp. 261–264, 2003.
[12] A. L. Wani, S. A. Bhat, and A. Ara, 'Omega-3 fatty acids and the treatment of depression: a review of scientific evidence,' Integr. Med. Res., vol. 4, no. 3, pp. 132–141, 2015.
[13] & M. Hendrix, Abernethy, Sloane, Misuraca, '基因的改变NIH Public Access,' Bone, vol. 23, no. 1, pp. 1–7, 2013.
[14] W. G. van Ginkel et al., 'The effect of various doses of phenylalanine supplementation on blood phenylalanine and tyrosine concentrations in tyrosinemia type 1 patients,' Nutrients, vol. 11, no. 11, pp. 1–11, 2019.
[15] Thorne Research Inc., 'Biotin Introduction,' Altern. Med. Rev., vol. 12, no. 1, pp. 73–78, 2007.
[16] S. Parker, P. Hanrahan, and C. Barrett, 'Folate for therapy,' Aust. Prescr., vol. 36, no. 2, pp. 52–55, 2013.
[17] G. Ball, 'Niacin: Nicotinic Acid and Nicotinamide,' Vitam. Their Role Hum. Body, pp. 1–18, 2004.
[18] G. S. Kelly, 'MONOGRAPHS Pantothenic Acid,' vol. 16, no. 3, 2011.
[19] P. Ch et al., 'Pyridoxine & Pyridoxal 5 ' Phosphate,' Altern. Med., vol. 6, no. 1, pp. 87–92, 2001.
[20] 'Copyright©2003 Thorne Research, Inc. All Rights Reserved. No Reprint Without Written Permission,' Altern. Med. Rev., vol. 8, no. 1, pp. 59–62, 2003.
[21] U. Gröber, J. Schmidt, and K. Kisters, 'Magnesium in prevention and therapy,' Nutrients, vol. 7, no. 9, pp. 8199–8226, 2015.
[22] H. Haase, S. Overbeck, and L. Rink, 'Zinc supplementation for the treatment or prevention of disease: Current status and future perspectives,' Exp. Gerontol., vol. 43, no. 5, pp. 394–408, 2008.
[23] I. N. Name, B. A. Name, and U. S. A. Name, 'Submission for Selenium,' pp. 1–13.

Solitude

Laugh, and the world laughs with you;
Weep, and you weep alone;
For the sad old earth must borrow its mirth,
But has trouble enough of its own.
Sing, and the hills will answer;
Sigh, it is lost on the air;
The echoes bound to a joyful sound,
But shrink from voicing care.
Rejoice, and men will seek you;
Grieve, and they turn and go;
They want full measure of all your pleasure,
But they do not need your woe.
Be glad, and your friends are many;
Be sad, and you lose them all,
There are none to decline your nectared wine,
But alone you must drink life's gall.
Feast, and your halls are crowded;
Fast, and the world goes by.
Succeed and give, and it helps you live,
But no man can help you die.
There is room in the halls of pleasure
For a large and lordly train,
But one by one we must all file on
Through the narrow aisles of pain.

by Ella Wheeler Wilcox

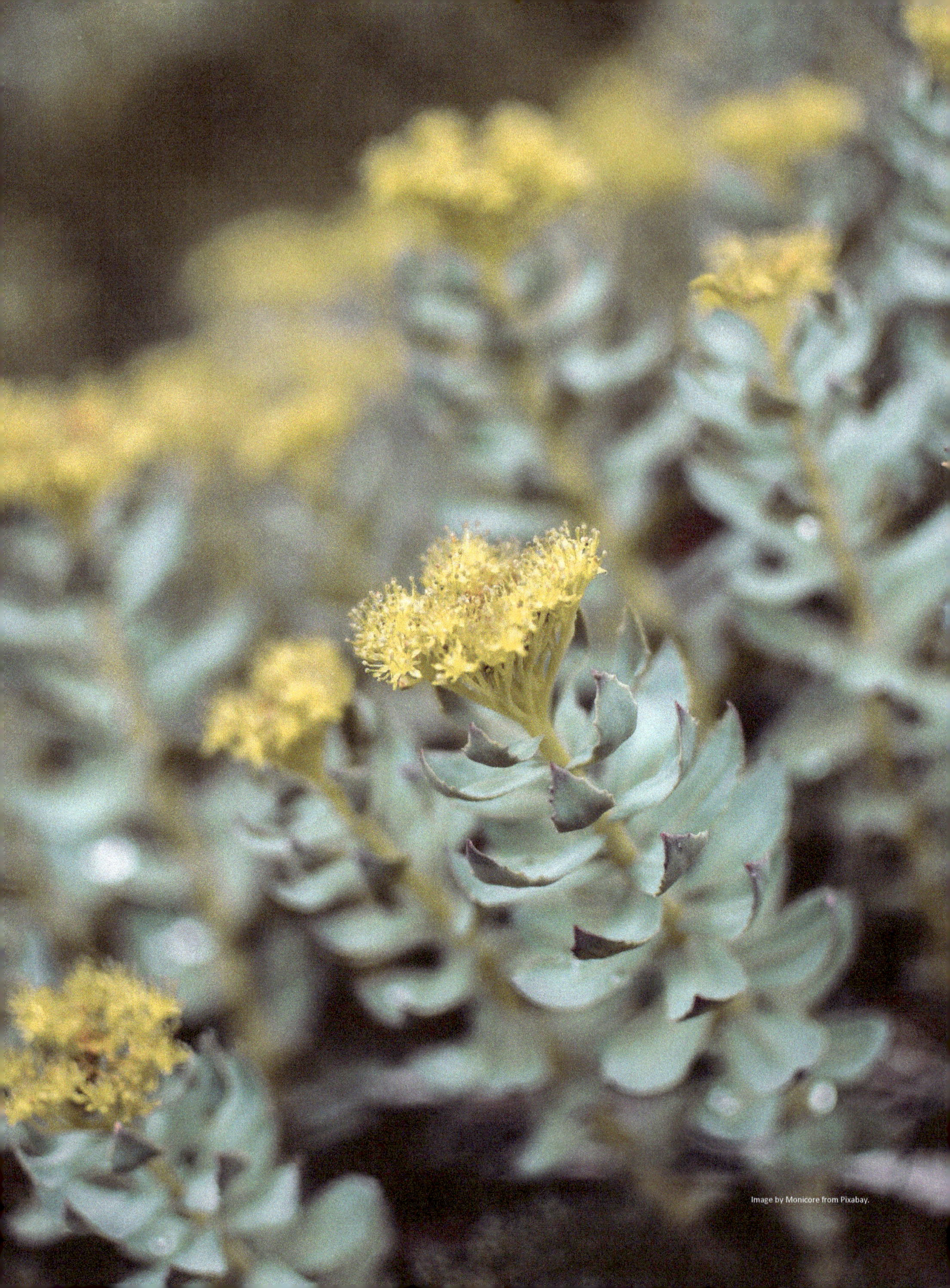

Image by Monicore from Pixabay.

Golden root - Rhodiola rosea

Known as Golden root or Arctic root, it is one of the few herbs in this book that grows predominantly in alpine regions in the northern hemisphere of Europe, Asia and America. It has long been used by the Russian, Scandinavian, Northern American and Chinese indigenous people. It was written about by Dioscorides in the first century. This herb may be considered the Northern Ginseng as it is viewed as an adaptogen in much the same way that Siberian Ginseng and Chinese Ginseng are. Within the research on this herb, there are consistent cautions on its use as it may interact with pharmaceutical antidepressants and have minor side effects such as nausea, agitation, restlessness and insomnia. Yet conversely, other sources indicate that the herb has little or no effectiveness in the treatment of health conditions. Such counterclaims add to the confusion that consumers may have in selecting an herbal supplement. If as stated the herb has side effects, one of which is Serotonin Syndrome, or the acute increase in serotonin levels, then such warnings in effect add to the support that the herb does have an influence on the body and is therefore effective if used wisely.

Rhodiola has been researched since the 1960s with much of this research occurring in Russia. It is believed that as an adaptogen it aids in the management of stress and associated side effects thereof. It has been recommended for increasing performance and stamina and has been advocated for use in the treatment of chronic fatigue syndrome. Other claims for the herb are that it improves mental acuity and focus, and that it acts as an antidepressant via its modulation of central stress response mechanisms through its effect on central neurotransmission and neuroendocrine function.

A study from the University of Pennsylvania, Philadelphia in 2015 sought to understand the role Rhodiola played in the alleviation of depressive-like symptoms. In this study, the herb was compared to the standard antidepressant known as sertraline, which is a selective serotonin reuptake inhibitor class of antidepressants. The researchers focused on Major Depressive Disorder (MDD) and used a target group of 48 individuals. The study concluded that 'Although R. rosea produced less antidepressant effect versus sertraline, it also resulted in significantly fewer adverse events and was better tolerated'. These findings suggest that R. rosea, although less effective than sertraline, may possess a more favourable risk to benefit ratio for individuals with mild to moderate depression.

A review of scientific research papers into the mood-altering actions of Rhodiola was carried out in 2016. This review also concluded there was substance to the claims that the herb alleviates depressive-like symptoms via the main compound found in the roots of the plant known as salidroside. Other vital compounds found in the plant's roots are tyrosol, rosavin and rhodioloside.

When considering this herb, the complete suite of health claims should be considered. Such aspects as aiding in the management of stress and anxiety. The improvement in mental health function is an attractive adjunct in an antidepressant herb. Yet as the literature for this particular plant stresses; please consult your physician or doctor before using it.

[1] J. J Mao, "Rhodiola Rosea Therapy for Major Depressive Disorder: A Study Protocol for a Randomized, Double-Blind, Placebo- Controlled Trial," J. Clin. Trials, vol. 04, no. 03, 2014.

[2] "Изучение индивидуальной изменчивости растений Rhodiola rosea L. в целях отбора ценных генотипов для микроклонального размножения," Известия Самарского Научного Центра Российской Академии Наук, vol. 15, no. 3–2. 2013.

[3] "Dangers of Rhodiola Rosea, ." .J. J. Mao et al., "Rhodiola rosea versus sertraline for major depressive disorder: A randomized placebo-controlled trial," Phytomedicine, vol. 22, no. 3, pp. 394–399, 2015.

[4] N. America and U. S. Food, "Rhodiola rosea," Altern. Med. Rev., vol. 7, no. 5, pp. 421–423, 2002.

[5] MHA, "Complementary & Alternative Medicine for Mental Health," p. 272, 2016.

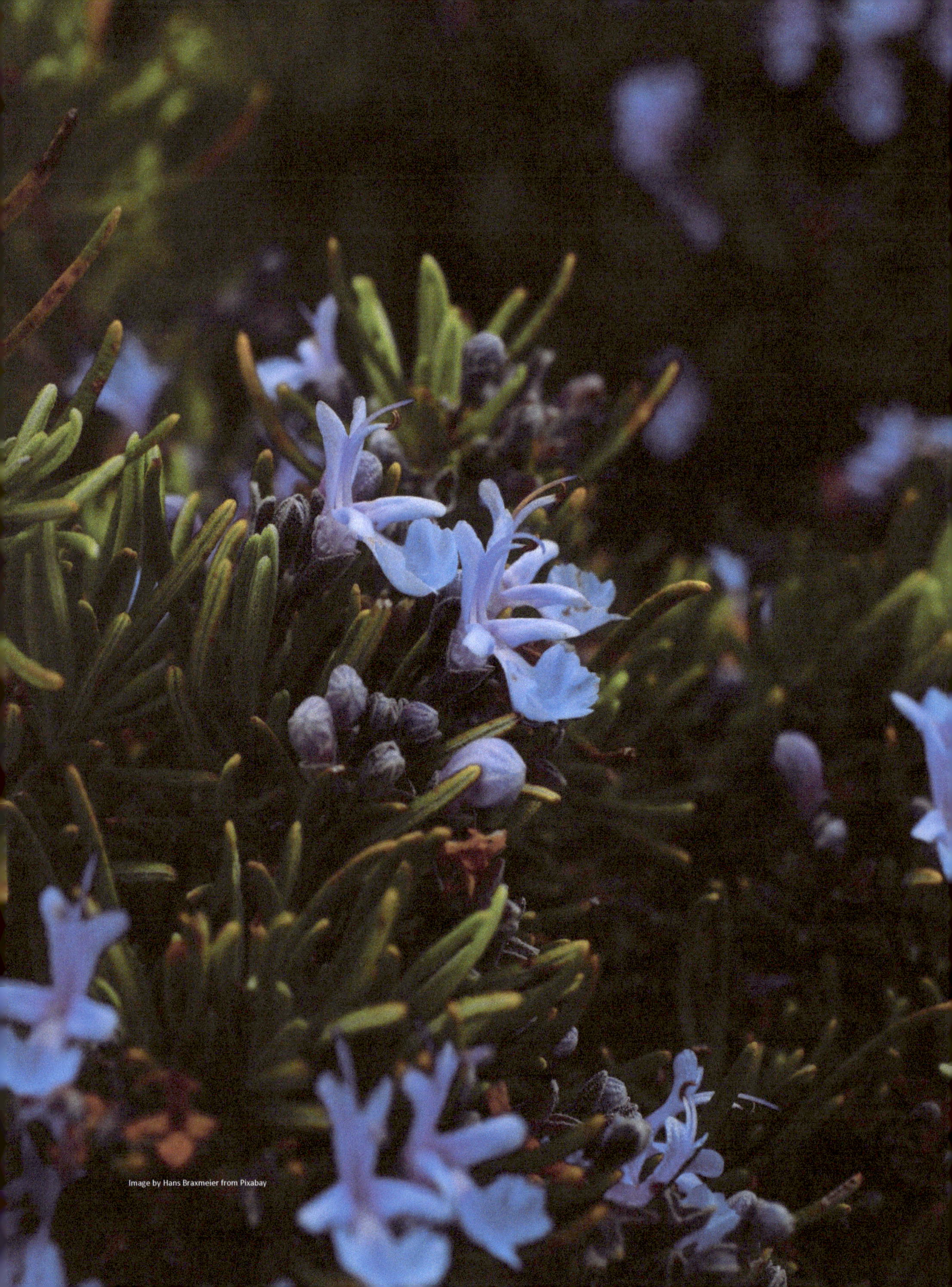
Image by Hans Braxmeier from Pixabay

Rosemary - Salvia rosmarinus

We all know Rosemary, but few know all her secrets. Rosemary has been around for a long, long time, from the birth of Aphrodite, when the herb was draped all around the emerging goddess, to cuneiform tablets from 5,000 years ago. As a result, it is woven throughout our histories and mythology. The name of the herb is thought to come from ancient Greek and Latin and is translated as 'dew of the sea' as it grew along the coastlines of the Mediterranean. The flowers were thought to be white until the Virgin Mary threw her cloak over a bush and the flowers turned blue. The herb is associated with love, remembrance, intellect, and is a ward against evil spirits. So, our standard culinary herb is packed with flavour and history. In 2017, Rosemary's scientific name was changed from Rosmarinus officinalis to Salvia Rosmarinus.

Not surprisingly Rosemary has been the focus of many scientific studies into its reported health benefits. Clinical findings have shown that the herb has antimicrobial, anti-inflammatory, anticancer, neuroprotective, antioxidant, antispasmodic, hepatoprotective and antidepressant actions. In short, the herb can be used as a general tonic for overall health. Yet, our focus is on the antidepressant findings.

The main compounds found in Rosemary are luteolin, carnosic acid, carnosol, betulinic acid, ursolic acid, and rosmarinic acid. In a research paper (2013) the researchers mention that several of these compounds are known to 'upregulate' two significant genes known as tyrosine hydroxylase and pyruvate carboxylase. They are involved in the regulations of dopaminergic, serotonergic and GABAergic pathway (gamma-aminobutyric acid (GABA)). As such, the use of rosemary (in this case the water extract) influences the monoaminergic system of serotonin, dopamine and the GABAergic pathway. The findings from this research showed that the aqueous extract at a dose of either 15 mg/kg or 30 mg/kg body weight outperformed the standard antidepressant drug imipramine.

Research into the anti-anxiety effects of Rosemary was carried out in 2016 at the Shahrekord University of Medical Sciences in Iran. The findings from this undertaking supported the use of the ethanol/aqueous extract of rosemary in the treatment of anxiety. The recommended doses used in this trial were 400 mg/kg body weight.

Many other trials and tests have been carried out on the claims that Rosemary is useful in the management of depression and anxiety. Yet, the claims that rosemary will actually improve memory has also been widely researched, and one study from the United Kingdom (2016) resulted in findings that strongly supported the use of rosemary in the treatment of dementia, especially Alzheimer's disease. Further research into such claims was carried out in 2017 and focused on another compound found in rosemary known as nepitrin. In this study it was found that this unique compound had similar actions to the standard drug donepezil, which is used in the treatment of Alzheimer's disease.

Therefore, Rosemary is not only highly effective in the treatment of depression and anxiety, but also useful in brain function and protection.

[1] Machado DG, Bettio LEB, Cunha MP, Capra JC, Dalmarco JB, et al. (2009) Antidepressant-like effect of the extract of Rosmarinus officinalis in mice: Involvement of the monoaminergic system. Progress in Neuro-Psychopharmacology & Biological Psychiatry 33: 642-650.

[2] Sasaki K, Omri AE, Kondo S, Han J, Isoda H (2013) Rosmarinus officinalis polyphenols produce antidepressant like effect through monoaminergic and cholinergic functions modulation. Behavioral Brain Research 238: 86-94.

[3] Machado DG, Cunha MP, Neis VB, Balen GO, Colla A, et al. (2013) Antidepressant-like effects of fractions, essential oil, carnosol and betulinic acid isolated from Rosmarinus officinalis L. Food Chemistry 136: 999-1005.

[4] Machado DG, Cunha MP, Neis VB, Balen GO, Colla AR, et al. (2012) Rosmarinus officinalis L. hydroalcoholic extract, similar to fluoxetine, reverses depressive-like behavior without altering learning deficit in olfactory bulbectomized mice. Journal of Ethnopharmacology 143: 158-169.

Soundtracks for depression

"The function of music is to release us from the tyranny of conscious thought!"

Thomas Beecham

The universe ebbs and flows to patterns and cycles that regulate all life. The patterns are studied by zealous physicists and over the last few centuries, these mad scientists poked, prodded, explored, laboured, and have thrown billions of dollars at these no longer secrets of our universe. From Pythagorean theory to Newton's three laws giving way to Plank's constant, and then supporting Einstein's theory of relativity on to the Berkenstein-Hawkin equation, and countless other voyagers of the universe who never left home or the lab. We have gained a better understanding of our position in this vast cosmos. The trajectories of planets and the oscillations of subatomic quarks and phasers have been studied and understood. Everything has its signature pattern and behaviour. There is a rhythm to life, and for us at the beginning of our lives, the most important rhythm we bind to is the beating hearts of our mothers, the first primal music.

In all cultures, in all corners of our world, music has always been with us. From the cave in Central Europe to the Serengeti of Africa our ancestors at first used percussion and voice in attempts to harness the secrets of rhythm and patterns. Perhaps it is our subconscious need for control, or maybe it is simply the art of creating comfort in trying to make sense of it all. Music has always been our highly prized way of interpreting life through sound.

Today we have moved from simple sticks, such as the Australian aboriginal clapping sticks, to computers in synthesizers. A lonely troubadour is now joined by symphony orchestras. The audience of a few around a lonely fire is now tens of thousands in sports arenas. We worship music like never before and have a plethora of genres and styles within it. From the elevator music of shopping malls and the soundtracks in our movies we are inundated by sound, and we love it. Yet some say silence is the only true sound of the soul, and meditations in the wilderness are now sought after by explorers of the spirit.

The mind as we are discussing here, is layered with memories of places, people and sounds. A piece of music, a simple song can bring back rainbows of the past as no other trigger can. A romance, a family gathering, a face is more often than not linked to soundtracks in our minds. As a result, it comes as no surprise that Music Therapy has earned its place in the therapeutic jungle of our modern-day life.

The pioneers of Music Therapy Peter Nordoff (1909-1977) and Clive Robbins (1927-2011) joined forces in the mid-twentieth century to explore and develop music as a therapeutic tool for children with special needs. In the same period Carl Orff (1895-1982) and Helen Lindquist Bonny (1921-2010) each in their own way developed strings to the modern therapy of music. Perhaps the most influential was the collaboration which became known as the Nordoff-Robbins music therapy and which has thousands of registered practitioners working today.

These practitioners work with all manner of psychiatric, physical and emotional issues. From autistic children to catatonic patients. Music has been shown to be a powerful adjunct to the health system, and the benefits from it are many. One such intriguing aspect is the use of music to make Alzheimer's patients remember events in their lives where for all intents and purposes they appear to have forgotten even the faces of their children. Parkinson's disease is also significantly ameliorated with Music Therapy where movement, memory and balance are all improved.

So, is it the music or the rhythm? Is it the pattern or the association with time? Or are all these involved in making music such a powerful therapeutic agent? Perhaps there is no need to know why, and simply accept the solid evidence that music is a powerful tool and that it has a profound effect on depression - which in some cases is however not for the better.

Left to our own devices we find that sometimes we make bad decisions, and for some people this is more common than for others. Therefore, for most people listening to music it is beneficial and either uplifting or at least comforting. Conversely, when we choose music that reinforces our negative thoughts, we have come to the point where it creates an environment 'conditioned' to the negative. In clinical hypnotherapy, the brain or mind's ability to absorb subliminal messages is well understood and utilised. This is exactly the same when we go about our daily lives with a soundtrack in the background. When we drive our cars, we focus on the skill of driving whilst the music from the sound system is allowed to penetrate into our subconscious minds unfiltered. If the music is negative, then this will have a consequential effect on our moods and how we view life.

As we travel through our daily lives, corporations, political parties, or religions all try to influence us in any way they can, and one of these is via the use of music. Studies have shown that people purchase more expensive wines in wine shops if classical music is playing. Other studies have shown we purchase more depending on the background music in shopping malls, and the use of patriotic stirring music is the bread and butter of political elections. So, we can safely say, if music has been used effectively in the marketplace to control us, then the correct use of music can and will reduce our anxiety and depression. However, we must choose our music wisely.

Choosing people and environments more often than not tends to suit our preconceived ideas. In our current period of the internet and social media, this is even more amplified due to the algorithms developed by various platforms such as Twitter or Facebook that refine the content to a point where the viewer only gets to see what is matched to their desires and perceptions. Any opposing views are filtered out. Elections and the periods prior to them are particularly disturbing as voters believe that they are the majority simply because they only see content that supports their point of view.

It is the same with music. When we are in our depressive funks, we tend to listen to music that fits our dark and dismal thoughts. There have even been various studies into what might be the best music to have at your funeral, with one finding the music from the Estonian composer Arvo Part by far the most popular composer for those final farewells. I am not sure as to whether Mr Part is pleased by such an accolade.

What is the right music to choose to lift our spirits? We all have differing tastes as a result of our cultures, religions, age, language, and experiences. Many studies have been conducted on the effects of different genres of music on mood and happiness, however, there are aspects within each individual that render these studies mere generalisations at best. They do supply us with information to help us choose wisely however.

New Age music might be the choice of one person and completely irritate another person. Classical music has been shown to improve the mood of mature people and did not elevate the moods of teens or young adults. Yet, Classical music is a broad genre and has all manner of pieces from Mozart's

Requiem to Schubert's Ave Maria, some are light and others dark. There appears to be a wealth of scientific literature on the damaging effects of Heavy Rock music (Grunge, Emo, Punk, Metallic rock etc.) Yet this is primarily in regard to anxiety and depression. The debate as to whether this genre of Heavy Rock contributes to acts of violence has not been supported in research. In another piece of research, it was shown that listening to Heavy Metal music is actually an aid in processing anger and not the cause of it.

The emergence of these types of musical genres occurred in the 1980s and '90s perhaps out of the anger and frustration of the youth of the time. Needless to say, they have created a perpetual loop and not a solution to these feelings. Whilst they are an expression of anger at the system that throughout history the youths of society have railed against, the end result remains the residual feeling of anxiety and depression. If you are a devotee of this genre then it might be wise to have a holiday from it for a while. So, we must consider wisely when claiming one music genre is more effective than another in elevating moods.

Here is a question. Why are both balance and hearing combined into the same organ of the body?

In our singular cells of depression, we find it comforting to listen to music that 'matches' what we feel. In so doing we create a universal library of sad or depressing music. The advent of the American Blues whether it was from the mournful music of slaves or from Field Hollers, men and women cried out a musical rhythm to keep field workers, railway gangs, chain gangs, moving. Country and Western music filled with tragedy and unrequited love echoed in the empty hills of rural desolation. At the present time, we can find music in all genres from Rock to Folk that we can relate to in our ennui. These comforting musical interludes come and validate us, assures us that even though we might feel completely alone at least we have a soundtrack to synchronise to. Yet, rarely do they lift us out of our pits of despair. In a wonderful research paper titled "Misery Loves Company" it was shown that when we are in a sad or depressed mood, we choose music that suits our darkness. This paper also showed that ambiguous music was less effective than unambiguous music. Or to put it another way, we should choose music with a clear uplifting message.

So, what has science uncovered as to the best music to alleviate anxiety and depression? The answer is not clear, however common sense should prevail, and for each person the answer will be different. There are however some basic fundamentals of sound; a major scale is preferred to a minor scale, and a fast-moving piece of music in the major scale elicits happier emotions than a similar piece on a minor scale. Once again this is a general rule yet one to pay attention to when you choose your music today or as weird as it may sound let your mascot choose the music. You might be surprised and get an answer. As Emmylou Harris said "When there are dogs and music, people have a good time!"

[1] D. K. Antrim, 'Music therapy,' Music. Q., vol. 30, no. 4, pp. 409–420, 1944.
[2] M. Khan and A. Ajmal, 'Effect of Classical and Pop Music on Mood and Performance,' Int. J. Sci. Res. Publ., vol. 7, no. 12, pp. 905–911, 2017.
[3] G. R. Shafron and M. P. Karno, 'Heavy metal music and emotional dysphoria among listeners.,' Psychol. Pop. Media Cult., vol. 2, no. 2, pp. 74–85, 2013.
[4] L. Sharman and G. A. Dingle, 'Extreme metal music and anger processing,' Front. Hum. Neurosci., vol. 9, no. APR, pp. 1–11, 2015.
[5] P. G. Hunter, E. G. Schellenberg, and A. T. Griffith, 'Misery loves company: Mood-congruent emotional responding to music,' Emotion, vol. 11, no. 5, pp. 1068–1072, 2011.
[6] N. Ahmad, 'Impact of music on mood: empirical investigation,' J. Res. Humanit. Soc. Sci., vol. 5, no. November, pp. 98–101, 2015.

Play list for depression

"Paint It Black" — Rolling Stones
I see a red door and I want to paint it black/ No colours anymore I want them to turn black

"Sound and Vision" — David Bowie
Pale blinds drawn all day/Nothing to do, nothing to say/Blue blue

"Lithium" — Evanescence
I can't hold on to me/ Wonder what's wrong with me

"Creep" — Radiohead
I'm a creep, I'm a weirdo/ What the hell am I doing here?/ I don't belong here

"Breathe Me" — Sia
Ouch I have lost myself again/ and I am nowhere to be found/ I think that I might break

"Help" — The Beatles
Help me if you can I'm feeling down/ And I do appreciate you being 'round/ Help me get my feet back on the ground

"Both Sides Now" — Joni Mitchell
I've looked at life from both sides now/ From win and lose and still somehow/ It's life's illusions I recall/ I really don't know life at all

"Behind Blue Eyes" — The Who
No one bites back as hard/ On their anger/ None of of my pain and woe/ show through

"I Am I Said" — Neil Diamond
I am, I said/ To no one there/ And no one heard at all/ Not even the chair

"People Are Strange" — The Doors
People are strange when you're a stranger/ Faces look ugly when you're alone

"Everybody Hurts" — REM
If you're on your own/ In this life/ The days and nights are long/ When you think you've had too much/ Of this life/ To hang on

"This Depression" — Bruce Springsteen
Baby I've been down/ But never this down/ I've been lost/ But never this lost

"Fire and Rain" — James Taylor
I've seen fire and I've seen rain/ I've seen sunny days that I thought would never end/ I've seen lonely times when I could not find a friend

"A Day Without Me" — U2
Started a landslide in my ego/ Looked from the outside to the world I left behind

"Here Comes The Rain Again" — Eurythmics
Here comes the rain again/ Raining in my head like a tragedy/ Tearing me apart like a new emotion

"Mad World" — Tears for Fears
I find kinda funny, find it kinda sad/ dreams in which I'm dying are the best I've ever had

"Lullaby" — Nickelback
Please let me take you/ Out of the darkness and into the light

Songs & videos available from https://parade.com

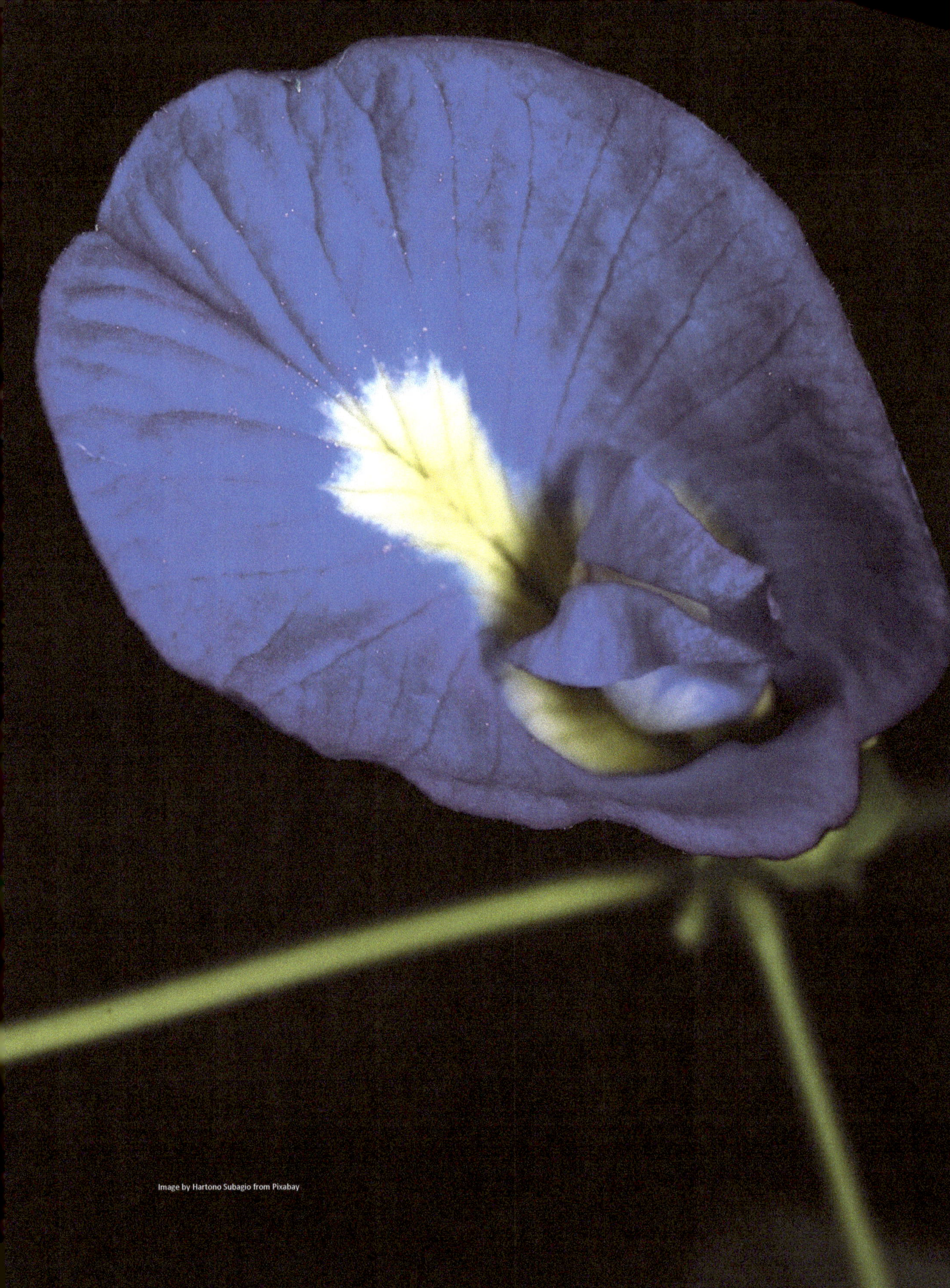

Image by Hartono Subagio from Pixabay

Asian Pigeonwings - Clitoria ternatea

Another name for the flower is Blue Pea or Butterfly Pea, making it easier to remember. One of the benefits of using this flower is that it has been shown to increase cognitive function and memory. And so not only will it lessen feelings of depression, but you will also become smarter.

It has been used for centuries in its native range tropical Asia. The flower is a staple, both as a food and medicine in Ayurvedic systems, Chinese, Malay and other nations of the region. The traditional claims of the benefits derived from using the Blue Pea flower are diuretic, anti-inflammatory, laxative, fever reducing, analgesic, antidiabetic, anxiolytic and anticonvulsant. Much of which has been studied in research from around the world. One caution should be noted for this herb is that it has also been traditionally used to induce miscarriage in pregnancy.

A widespread use of the plant is using the flowers to colour food and drinks. A unique feature is that in a neutral Ph liquid, such as water, the flowers make a mesmerising blue drink. However, if the Ph changes to a more acidic nature, the colour will change to a pinkish purple. In this way, it is currently being used in a gin brand to turn its gin from blue to a pink when tonic is added. The flowers are also used to turn rice blue in Malaysia. The aerial part of the plant (leaves and flowers) show anti-anxiety and anti-depression effects, it is the roots that are the most effective parts of the plant in this regard.

In a study conducted in 2013, it was shown that the root extract had a similar action when compared to the standard antidepressant drug, imipramine. In this research the root extract also compared favourably to the drug diazepam which is used to treat anxiety. Doses of 300 mg/kg body weight had the most desirable results.

A more recent review of trials done of the herb has further supported these claims. This paper reviewed approximately 92 articles and found that Blue Pea flowers and especially the roots are a powerful herb in the treatment of depression, anxiety and brain function. In citing one particular paper, researchers used the root extract (50 mg/body weight) in juvenile rats and found a permanent increase in brain function. The researchers believe that the extract increases the nerve growth factor (NGF), thereby improving the physiology of the brain in youth.

So, we can see that Clitoria ternatea is a beneficial herb in the treatment of depression, anxiety and nootropic (pronounced no-a-tropic) challenges. Nootropic simply means drugs that enhance the brain. Fortunately, the herb does not act as a sedative, and as a result, it may be thought of an emotional and intellectual tonic of significant importance.

Buying yourself a bottle of the blue gin might be an excellent way to attempt to treat your depression. However, the juniper in the gin might make you slow down as it acts as a soporific or in plain English, it makes you drowsy.

[1] M. Parvathi and K. Ravishankar, "Evaluation of antidepressant, motor coordination and locomotor activities of ethanolic root extract of Clitoria ternatea," J. Nat. Remedies, vol. 13, no. 1, pp. 19–24, 2013.

[2] J. Mehla, "Clitoria ternatea Linn: A herb with potential pharmacological activities: future Prospects as therapeutic herbal medicine," J. Pharmacol. Reports, vol. 3, no. 1, pp. 1–8, 2018.

[3] M. Chwil, R. Matraszek-Gawron, P. Terlecka, and M. Kostryco, "Plant antidepressants in selected species from the family Fabaceae – a review," Ann. Hortic., vol. 27, no. 3, pp. 57–68, 2018.

[4] S. S. Azimova and A. I. Glushenkova, "Clitoria ternatea," Lipids, Lipophilic Components Essent. Oils from Plant Sources, pp. 568–568, 2012.

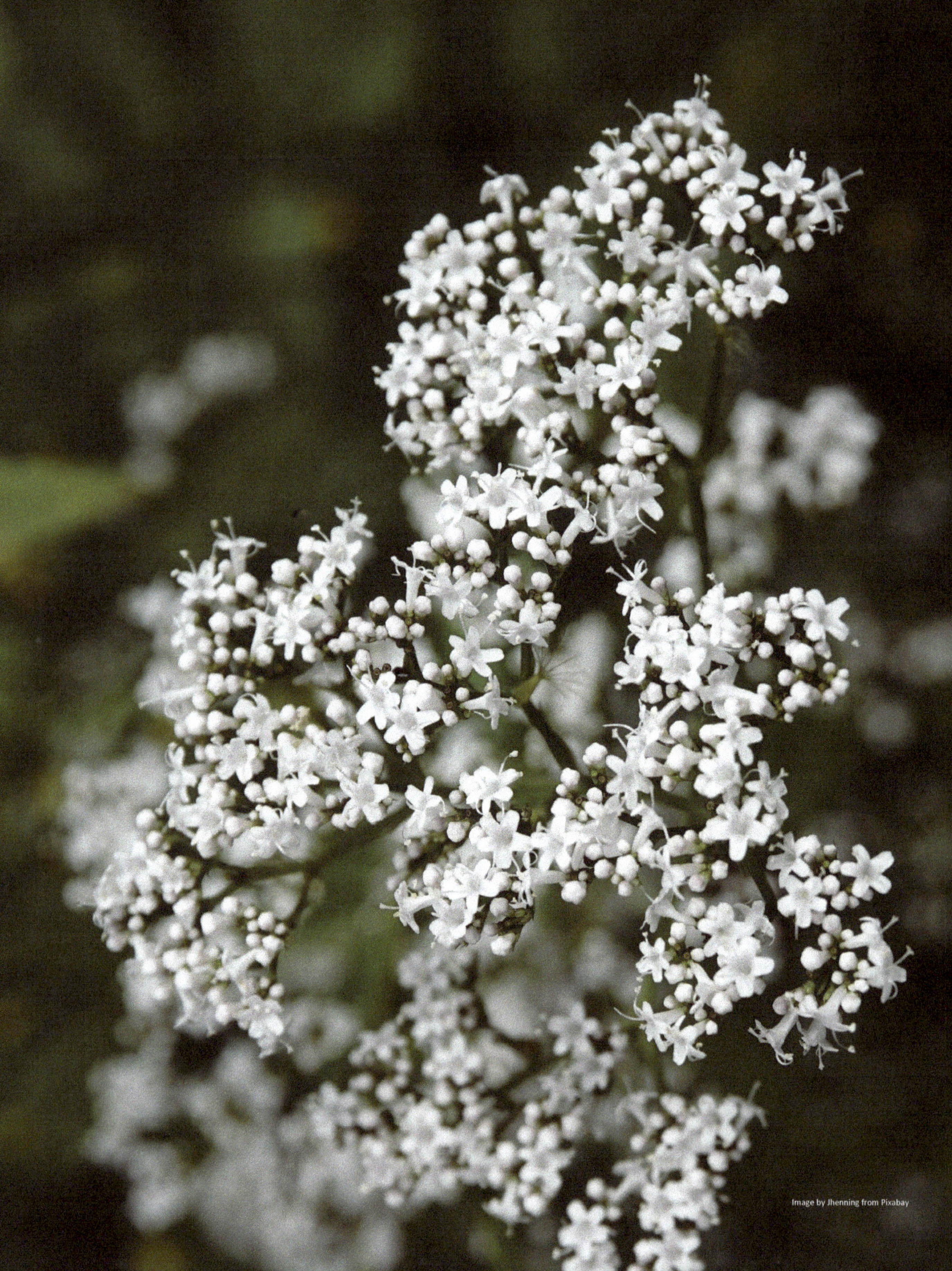

Image by Jhenning from Pixabay

Valerian - Valeriana officinalis

Valerian has been used since antiquity, and as such is referenced in Greek as well as Roman medicinal texts and grows throughout Europe. When the history of the use of valerian is studied it quickly becomes clear that it was one of the most important herbs throughout this region for centuries. As such it is woven into tales of mythology and religion. The roman Emperor Publius Lucinius Valerianus may have been after the plant. The name is derived from the Latin word 'valere' meaning 'to be strong and healthy, worth, to be valid, to count The Germanic goddess Hertha is reported to have used bunches of valerian to whip the oxen towing her cart and in Sweden the groom would wear bunches of valerian to ward off jealous elves when he was getting married. The herb is even mentioned in the books of Harry Potter. Not only was valerian used in sleeping potions, but it was also the main ingredient in love potions and in ancient Greece it was traditionally hung in windows to ward off evil spirits. In all a very useful herb with all manner of strange applications.

The flowers can be either white or pink and have been a staple in medieval diets. The plant may grow up to five feet/ two meters tall and display umbrellas of the white or pink flowers which can be used in wine or food. The active parts or medicinal parts of the plant are the roots which are best collected from plants that are over two years old in early autumn.

Relatives of valerian officinalis plant is also found in Asia and North America where they have also been used in the traditional medical systems that developed in these regions.

It was thought that Valerian was a sedative. However, this is not entirely correct as research from 2007 had findings showing that the extract from the roots of the plant did not relax muscles nor act as a sedative, but rather acted as an anti-anxiety or anxiolytic therapy. As a result, the unique compounds found in Valerian, being valeric acid, gamma-aminobutyric acid (GABA), valerene, valerianine and valepotriates, may act in a manner that influence monoamine synthesis, and as such relieve anxiety and depression. It is estimated that there may be more than 150 chemical compounds making up Valerian.

Valerian has been studied repeatedly for its sleep-inducing effects, and much of the research has endorsed its use for insomnia. The root extract has also been recommended for people who are coming off anti-anxiety medications because it softens the withdrawal symptoms.

Another study in 2009 found that the commercial preparation of valerian known as Phytofin Valerian 368 had a significant effect on the inhibition of noradrenaline reuptake, a mild effect on serotonin and no influence on dopamine synthesis. Yet an earlier report from 2003 stated that the root extract, and some compounds found in it, bind to the dopamine receptors. Another study from 2012 showed that the use of an ethanol based extract of its roots did have a significant effect on depression in test animals. Whilst this study did result in supporting the use of the plant, the researchers did admit that the precise manner in which this occurred is unclear. As a general rule, the positive effects will take one to two weeks to be felt. So, take your time when deciding if this herb is right for you. The recommended dose is thought to be between 450 to 600 mg/kg body weight, but it is still much debated.

Valerian is also used to treat convulsions, pain, hypertension, antiviral and angina. Studies have shown that valerian is non-toxic and therefore safe, however there are some studies that state the herb should not be taken during pregnancy.

On a more amusing note, the roots of the plant attract cats in much the same way that Catnip does. So, for all those depressed cat people out there, this herb may be ideal for you.

[1] H. Slomp Junior, G. Seniski, C. da Cunha, E. A. Audi, and R. Andreatini, "The combination of Passiflora alata and Valeriana officinalis on memory tasks in mice: Comparison with diazepam," Brazilian Arch. Biol. Technol., vol. 53, no. 6, pp. 1343–1350, 2010.

[2] B. Şen and A. Mat, "Chemical and medicinal evaluations of the Valeriana species in Turkey," J. Pharm. Istanbul Univ., vol. 45, no. 2, pp. 267–276, 2015.

[3] V. Jatamansil et al., "Valerian Monograph," Univ. Color. Denver, no. 1, pp. 3–6, 2003.

[4] B. Walbroel, B. Feistel, R. Lehnfeld, and K. Appel, "Antidepressant activity of a refined valerian extract – an interesting new feature," Zeitschrift für Phyther., vol. 29, no. S 1, pp. 2008–2009, 2008.

Grey rainbows

"Try to be a rainbow in someone else's cloud"

Maya Angelou

If the saying "The eyes are the windows to the soul" were to be true, then if the person were depressed, the windows would be very dim indeed. Colour and mood have been linked throughout our history, from cave paintings to street graffiti. We have used colours to convey meanings and emotions. In hospitals, factories, offices, and homes, we all carefully select colours that define work and family. In advertising, a colour is a critical tool in the goal of getting us to consume this product or that. So, it should come as no surprise that colour and our ability to see it can be dramatically impacted by depression.

We often say we are 'blue' when in a sad mood. As we have discussed, the mascot for depression is a black dog, and it's common to say that "the colours have gone from life" when we suffer loss and trauma. Now science has arrived at some very surprising outcomes that, as we have said before, are not really that surprising as depression has always been associated with lack of colour.

People who suffer vision loss, no matter whether rapid or slow, have a higher than average chance of entering a depression.

People who suffer from depression, no matter whether it is a major depressive syndrome or minor, have a higher than average chance of losing normal vision.

Both of these statements are true and herein lies another mystery about depression as it is unclear which comes first, vision loss or depression.

In a study conducted in 2013 of 10,480 people over the age of twenty, who were asked to rate their depression and whether they had issues with eyesight, the overwhelming outcome of this study was a clear link between loss of vision and the feeling of despair. Naturally, few people would think that losing their sight to be a happy thing. So, no surprises here. And not surprising either when a study into age-related macular degeneration in the elderly also found a direct correlation between depression and the gradual loss of vision. These studies focused on the aspect of vision loss and its impact on a person's mood. Yet in other research it has been found that depression will actually reduce the sufferer's ability to see colours and contrasts, and it may even be a factor in vision loss if left untreated over time.

In one study (2007) from the University of Freiburg, Germany the researchers sought to understand why the ability to see colour contrasts was diminished in people suffering from depression. The results supported the fact that people who suffered from depression had a lower ability to differentiate contrast of colours. One of the fascinating outcomes from this study was the fact that even if the subject was being treated with antidepressants, their ability to see contrasts was still diminished. The link between the neurotransmitter dopamine and colour sensitivity was highlighted in this research.

Dopamine had been studied for many years prior to 2007 as it was linked to the debilitating condition known as Parkinson's disease. It was long known that this disease is the result of neurons in the brain that produce dopamine become damaged or die and thereby creating a significant reduction in the levels of dopamine in the brain. In the study of the disease, the role of dopamine in the human body became more transparent highlighting the realisation of how vital dopamine is for eyesight and eye health. The retina of the eye is rich in dopamine, and the health of the eye is now permanently linked to this fact. It has been shown that direct sunlight stimulates the release of dopamine in the eye. Therefore, spending too much time indoors (in front of a computer screen) will have disastrous effects on our eye health. The role of dopamine is thought to be circadian in nature, helping us see contrasts and colour more clearly and even improving high spatial recognition during the day. Getting outside and soaking up the sun is not only beneficial for vitamin D synthesis, but also for increasing dopamine and by default your eyesight, and both will help with your depression.

Over 80% of the body's dopamine stores are found in the brain, making it the most concentrated neurotransmitter in this organ. Additional research into the role of dopamine in depressive states and the correlation with eyesight have resulted in many medical practitioners considering eye tests as a fundamental clinical tool in diagnosing depression.

Therefore, should a person be suffering from depression due to lowered neurotransmitters serotonin, norepinephrine and dopamine, their eyesight will also be affected, and this then supports the long tradition of equating lack of colours in a depressing world.

In a more recent study a more worrying statistic was highlighted, that of the growing epidemic of myopia in the global youth. It has been estimated that almost 2.5 billion people will suffer from myopia, the inability to see distances clearly, with the majority of the youth in China and South Korea being the most concentrated sufferers at 95% of the youthful population. This research focused purely on the role of dopamine and its lack in the rise of myopia. The worrying part of this research is that the numbers almost mirror the emerging prevalence or growth of depression.

Sadly, dopamine cannot cross the blood-brain barrier, which makes supplements or injection of the neurotransmitter almost useless in treating depression because it will not get to where it is needed the most. Yet, the building blocks of dopamine can have a beneficial effect. The amino acid tyrosine is one of the main building blocks that the body synthesises dopamine from. Fortunately, tyrosine is not considered to be an essential mineral as there is so much of it in our environment that we rarely have a deficit in our bodies, and we can also make it ourselves. Yet, an essential amino acid phenylalanine is required to make tyrosine. Are you confused yet? Allow me to explain. Our bodies can produce our own tyrosine from phenylalanine which we can't produce. Therefore, we need to consume phenylalanine from our food. Hence it is considered to be an essential amino acid. Phenylalanine is found in the breast milk of mammals as well as eggs, beef, soybeans and some other food sources. At any rate, both phenylalanine and tyrosine can pass easily through the blood-brain barrier and can be synthesised into dopamine in the brain directly. The other important piece of information is that the other neurotransmitter norepinephrine is synthesised from dopamine, so a deficit in dopamine will not merely affect your eyes but also your mood as two of the main monoamines you need to be happy will be reduced. Dopamine, and the lack of it, is considered to be the cause of anhedonia or the lack of finding pleasure in anything.

Now if things aren't bad enough, what with the dimming of our colours and light. It has been found in associated research that depressed people will actually go out and make things worse by choosing the entirely wrong colours. Ever since Dr Max Luscher developed the first colour personality test in

1947 we have been messing around with colour therapy to varying degrees of success. It is no surprise that there are proponents of it and detractors, once again. All we can say is that ever since the first Neanderthal had a down day and refused to come out of his or her cave, preferring to be alone and paint pretty pictures on the wall, we have associated colours with our moods. As we can see from the research into depression and vision, our ability to see colours is affected, and therefore any claim that colour therapy is not effective is simply wrong. A quick search across scientific journals and reports will turn up countless studies into the best colour for hospital wards and psychiatric wards. One such paper from 2016 is an excellent example of this desire to improve the emotional environment in hospital wards for children by defining the most appropriate colour schemes.

A research paper into the most common colours chosen by people who suffer from anxiety, depression and impulsivity, found that people who suffer from depression prefer the colour grey whilst people suffering from anxiety chose black. People who are impulsive risk-takers chose yellow or red. Hence, we can see how depressive people work to keep themselves in their dungeons by decorating them with cold, lifeless choices such as grey and black. It is understood that a choice in music, colour, smell, food, and friends will either help to free you or imprison you. It's your choice, but hopefully, you will choose wisely.

Blue was defined by Dr Luscher as imparting calmness, tenderness, and tranquillity. Brown was defined as imparting an awareness of your own body with green being persistence, self-esteem, and pride. So, these colours would be a better choice. Choosing yellow whilst contentious as people either love it or hate, would impart the sense of exhilaration, activeness, and aspirations. On the other hand, you could stay with black, which according to the good doctor imparts emptiness and surrender, or grey that will help you withdraw and not be involved. As said, your choice. Although a new more colourful wardrobe may be a powerful tonic for your low moods

Colour therapy is of course integral to art therapy, especially if a painting is an artistic pursuit. It is relatively easy to look at a painting and assume the artist was either happy or sad at the time they made it by analysing its colours. If you have not seen Edvard Munch's famous painting known as "The Scream" with its cold colours of grey and black overhung with violent reds, then perhaps have a look at one man's impression of anxiety and check it out. He later described his inspiration for the painting by saying "I was walking along the road with two friends – the sun was setting – suddenly the sky turned blood red – I paused, feeling exhausted, and leaned on the fence – there were blood and tongues of fire above the blue-black fjord and the city – my friends walked on, and I stood there trembling with anxiety – and I sensed an infinite scream passing through nature".

Your dog doesn't care what colour you wear just that you love relentlessly. Why not paint the doghouse a bright colour today?

[1] K. Y. H. Pratik K. Mutha, Robert L. Sainburg, '基因的改变NIH Public Access,' Bone, vol. 23, no. 1, pp. 1–7, 2008.

[2] B. W. Rovner, R. J. Casten, and W. S. Tasman, 'Effect of depression on vision function in age-related macular degeneration,' Arch. Ophthalmol., vol. 120, no. 8, pp. 1041–1044, 2002.

[3] E. Bubl, L. Tebartz Van Elst, M. Gondan, D. Ebert, and M. W. Greenlee, 'Vision in depressive disorder,' World J. Biol. Psychiatry, vol. 10, no. 4 PART 2, pp. 377–384, 2009.

[4] X. Zhou, M. T. Pardue, P. M. Iuvone, and J. Qu, 'Dopamine signaling and myopia development: What are the key challenges,' Prog. Retin. Eye Res., vol. 61, pp. 60–71, 2017.

[5] C. R. Jackson et al., 'Retinal dopamine mediates multiple dimensions of light-adapted vision,' J. Neurosci., vol. 32, no. 27, pp. 9359–9368, 2012.

[6] L. Khodakhah Jeddi, 'The Analysis of Effect of Colour Psychology on Environmental Graphic in Children Ward at Medical Centres,' Psychol. Behav. Sci., vol. 5, no. 2, p. 51, 2016.

[7] S. Korkmaz, Ö. Özer, Ş. Kaya, A. Kazgan, and M. Atmaca, 'The correlation between color choices and impulsivity, anxiety and depression,' Eur. J. Gen. Med., vol. 13, no. 3, pp. 47–50, 2016.

Colour therapy

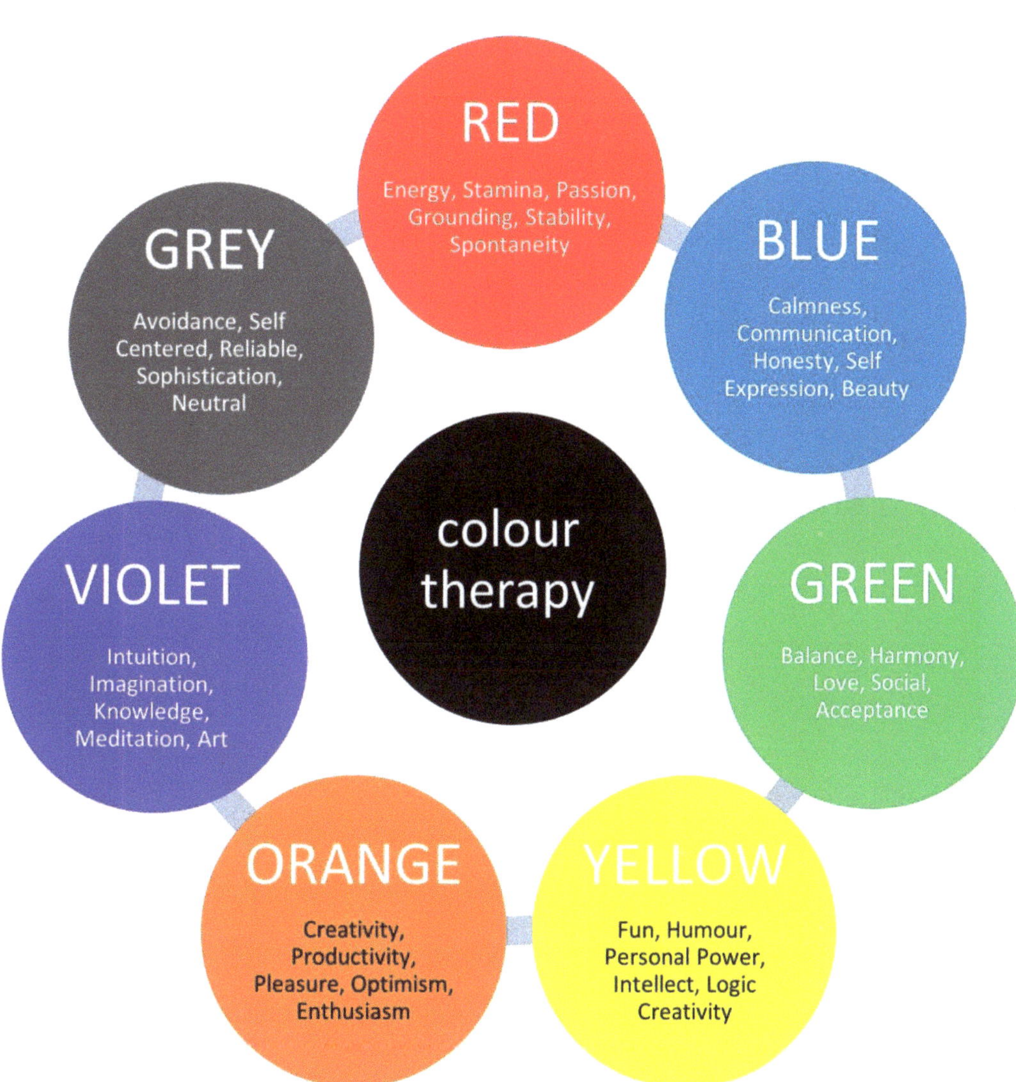
RED
Energy, Stamina, Passion, Grounding, Stability, Spontaneity
BLUE
Calmness, Communication, Honesty, Self Expression, Beauty
GREEN
Balance, Harmony, Love, Social, Acceptance
YELLOW
Fun, Humour, Personal Power, Intellect, Logic Creativity
ORANGE
Creativity, Productivity, Pleasure, Optimism, Enthusiasm
VIOLET
Intuition, Imagination, Knowledge, Meditation, Art
GREY
Avoidance, Self Centered, Reliable, Sophistication, Neutral
colour therapy

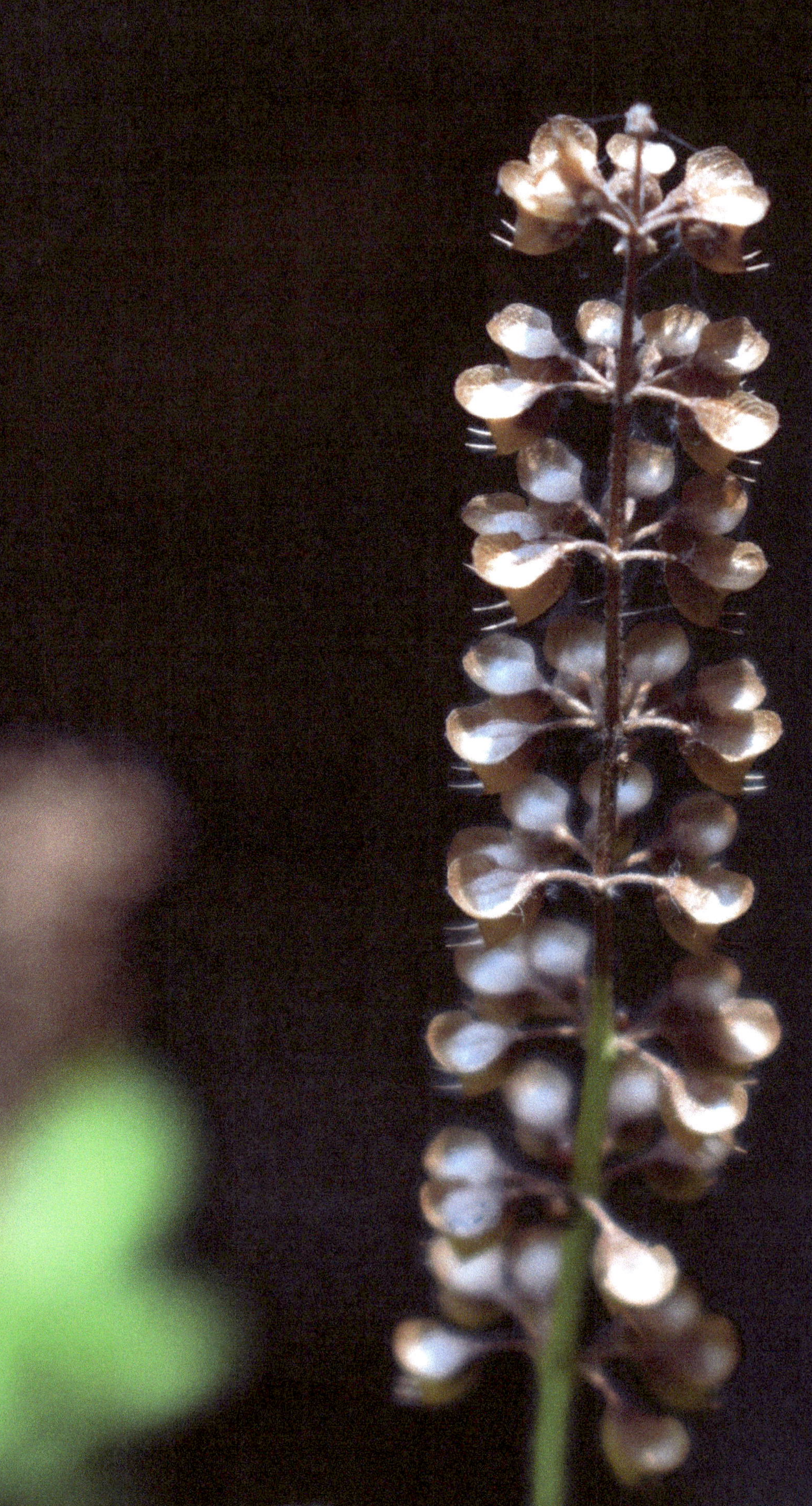

Image by Sandeep Hand from Pixabay

Tulsi - Ocimum sanctum

Tulsi has been claimed to be one of India's most important herbs. It has been used for thousands of years in Ayurvedic medicine and Unani medical systems. The plant has various other names, one of which is Holy Basil due to its importance in the religious ceremonies and devotions of the Hindu religion. The plant is associated with Vishnu, and Hindus believe that the goddess Lakshmi resides within the plant. It is commonly planted outside temples to Haruman and other Gods of the Hindu pantheon.

Claims that Tulsi is an adaptogen (a medicine considered to be a general tonic explicitly aiding in the management of stress) has been supported in clinical research, and therefore the herb may be viewed as similar to Ginseng and Siberian Ginseng in its usage. Research from 2014 sought to compare the antidepressant actions of the ethanol extract from its leaves to the standard antidepressant drug imipramine. The researchers found that over a 15 day period where the test animals were given an 8 mg/kg body weight dose, the results showed that Tulsi was as effective as imipramine.

The essential oil from the leaves of the Tulsi plant was studied in 2015 for its ability to reduce anxiety and depression. In this research the simple inhalation of the essential oil showed a significant decrease in symptoms, and that was supported in the claims that wearing the oil or having a diffuser in a home setting is useful in managing depression and anxiety. The main compounds found in the oil were linalool, camphor, β-elemene, α-bergamotene and bornyl-acetate, estragole, eugenol and 8-cineole.

An older study from 2007 employed 35 volunteers to undergo testing as to the efficacy of Tulsi in the reduction of stress and depression over 60 days. All volunteers were diagnosed with Generalised Anxiety Disorder (GAD), and the average age of the participants was 38 years old, with an age range of 16 to 60 years. The findings from this study showed that using doses of 500 mg equivalent of the herb twice daily resulted in an average of 30% reduction in stress, anxiety and depression over the period with an increase of 30% in attentive attitudes.

In other research and clinical testing, the herb has been shown to have antibacterial properties and immunostimulants. In addition to these, the herb has been shown to have anti-inflammatory action, which would aid in the treatment of depression. One of the main compounds found within the plant is known as eugenol. Eugenol has pain reduction and anaesthetic like properties, and this indicates the central nervous system relaxant aspects of the plant.

[1] G. Manu, N. G. Hema, and B. M. Parashivamurthy, Study of correlation of antidepressive effects of ethanolic leaf extract of Ocimum Ocimum sanctum and imipramine in albino mice, vol. 13, no. January, pp. 472–477, 2015.

[2] I. Tabassum, Z. N. Siddiqui, and S. J. Rizvi, "Effects of Ocimum sanctum and Camellia sinensis on stress-induced anxiety and depression in male albino Rattus norvegicus," Indian J. Pharmacol., vol. 42, no. 5, pp. 283–288, 2010.

[3] R. K. Verma, "In Vivo Evaluation of the Antidepressant Activity of a Novel Polyherbal Formulation," Autism. Open. Access, vol. 6, no. 4, 2016.

[4] S. Asian et al., "Ocimum tenuiflorum."

[5] D. Bhattacharyya, T. K. Sur, U. Jana, and P. K. Debnath, "Controlled programmed trial of Ocimum sanctum leaf on generalized anxiety disorders.," Nepal Med. Coll. J., vol. 10, no. 3, pp. 176–179, 2008.

A touchstone

"Touch comes before sight, before speech.
It is the first language and the last and it always tells the truth"

Margaret Atwood

The definition of a 'touchstone' is defined firstly as "A *fundamental part or feature to describe a comparison with*", or in the other definition *"It is a stone that was used to test the purity of gold or silver"*. Whichever definition you would like to use they both apply when we discuss the importance of human touch in the context of depressions and darkness.

Of the five senses touch may be considered the most fundamental upon which the other four rely. It is the first of the sensations we experience in the womb. Throughout life it is the basis of our secret yearnings and illicit dreams of where and how to be touched. However, it is also the first sense we disconnect entering into the world of depression. Either we believe that we are not good enough to be touched, or we do not wish to feel connected to others.

The power of the human touch is surprising and considerable. Human touch of the skin affects various bodily functions, including the promotion of growth in premature babies. It aids in the improvement of respiration and the immune response, the reduction of blood pressure and heart rate, the decrease of adrenal catecholamine secretion, increase of spinal cord blood flow, and also pain control during labour. Tactile stimulation also produces psychological effects such as relaxation for the alleviation of anxiety and depression during labour. The touch from a person will also reduce a sense of fatigue, anxiety and mood disorders in patients with cancer. Many scientific papers have been written on the physical and psychological benefits of touch, and many of these have highlighted the reduction in the symptoms of depression.

One of the hall marks of depression is when the person suffering begins to isolate from others. Why? It is a slow gentle unnoticeable withdrawal in the beginning due to thoughts of inferiority or any other trigger. Depression is able to take a normal carefree child, and over time as they age make them fold into themselves, reducing them in posture and personality to a point where intimacy is shunned, and touch avoided.

In many cases depression comes to visit those who are already isolated by family and lack of friends. With these people touch and warmth were not a common staple in their lives and the lessons of how to love someone else let alone themselves were never conducted. Touch for these people is a rare gift, random in its affection and occurrence.

The casual hand on an arm or shoulder can work wonders over time. The intense innocent hug from a friend or family member can be powerful medicine, however it may need to be repeated often over several weeks until the patient is in a stable condition.

One of the mysteries about touch is that it flows in two ways. From the giver to the receiver and back again. As such, care should be exercised when utilising it. Ask any sports therapist or masseuse and they will agree that in their practice of healing muscles and bones it is often the case that the therapist will experience the same symptoms as the patient they are treating. Likewise, a touch may be the same as water to an unquenchable thirst and the receiver may try and take too much too quickly.

Touch is considered to be one of the non-verbal communications conduits, and as such has been shown to have a direct influence during conversations, especially where a power imbalance was seen. In research exploring the use of touch in married heterosexual couples, women were found to touch their partners during discussions more, especially when opposing points of view were being debated. Needless to say, women employed more methods to support their positions than men did, touch being one of these tools.

From the effect of a mother's touch on her baby to the hug given to a grandmother from her grandchildren, touch is universal to us all. Yet the mystery has not been solved as to what the mechanics are. Is it electrical, or chemical as in pheromones, or both? Is it spiritual? We simply do not know as yet, other than one human touching another in a beneficial and reciprocated manner has a multitude of positive outcomes.

Research has shown that animals, pets to be precise, lessen feelings of loneliness and loss. By including a cat or dog into a retirees home or cancer ward has resulted in enormous benefits for those living within them. An animal whether real or imagined as a simple companion may be all that is required to bring happiness back from wherever it retreated to. Your mascot your totem animal by default has power.

In only using words no matter whether words of love on support or undeniable logic the desired outcome is more assured if they are accompanied by touch. To try and help someone out of their depression you will have a much higher chance of success with a hug or a friendly hand on an arm. Conversely if you are the one depressed and find no one around you that you would feel comfortable asking for a hug, then randomly hugging strangers would be a bad life choice. However, science has shown a therapeutic massage is highly effective. And for those who like the less therapeutic type of massages, the science has also shown these to be effective as well.

Regardless, you have your mascot to keep in touch with.

[1] White JL, Labarba RC (1976) The effects of tactile and kinesthetic stimulation on neonatal development in the premature infant. Dev Psychobiol 9:569–577

[2] Field TM, Schanberg SM, Scafidi F, Bauer CR, Vega-Lahr N, Garcia R, Nystrom J, Kuhn CM (1986) Tactile/kinesthetic stimulation effects on preterm neonates. Pediatrics 77:654–658

[3] Mathai S, Fernandez A, Mondkar J, Kanbur W (2001) Effects of tactile-kinesthetic stimulation in preterms: a controlled trial. Indian Pediatr 38:1091–1098

[4] Rojas MA, Kaplan M, Quevedo M, Sherwonit E, Foster LB, Ehrenkranz RA, Mayes L (2003) Somatic growth of preterm infants during skin-to-skin care versus traditional holding: a randomized, controlled trial. J Dev Behav Pediatr 24:163–168

[5] Field T, Henteleff T, Hernandez-Reif M, Martinez E, Mavunda K, Kuhn C, Schanberg S (1998) Children with asthma have improved pulmonary functions after massage therapy. J Pediatr 132:854–858

[6] Ironson G, Field T, Scafidi F, Hashimoto M, Kumar M, Kumar A, Price A, Goncalves A, Burman I, Tetenman C, Patarca R, Fletcher MA (1996) Massage therapy is associated with enhancement of the immune system's cytotoxic capacity. Int J Neurosci 84:205–217

[7] Meek SS (1993) Effects of slow stroke back massage on relaxation in hospice clients. Image J Nurs Sch 25:17–21

[8] Kurosawa M, Lundeberg T, Agren G, Lund I, Uvnas-Moberg K (1995) Massage-like stroking of the abdomen lowers blood pressure in anesthetized rats: influence of oxytocin. J Auton Nerv Syst 56:26–30

[9] Lund I, Lundeberg T, Kurosawa M, Uvnas-Moberg K (1999) Sensory stimulation (massage) reduces blood pressure in unanaesthetized rats. J Auton Nerv Syst 78:30–37

[10] Araki T, Ito K, Kurosawa M, Sato A (1984) Responses of adrenal sympathetic nerve activity and catecholamine secretion to cutaneous stimulation in anesthetized rats. Neuroscience 12:289–299

[11] Araki T, Hamamoto T, Kurosawa M, Sato A (1980) Response of adrenal efferent nerve activity to noxious stimulation of the skin. Neurosci Lett 17:131–135

[12] Kurosawa M, Toda H, Watanabe O, Budgell B (2007) Contribution of supraspinal and spinal structures to the responses of dorsal spinal cord blood flow to innocuous cutaneous brushing in rats. Auton Neurosci 136:96–99

[13] Field T, Ironson G, Scafidi F, Nawrocki T, Goncalves A, Burman I, Pickens J, Fox N, Schanberg S, Kuhn C (1996) Massage therapy reduces anxiety and enhances EEG pattern of alertness and math computations. Int J Neurosci 86:197–205

[14] Post-White J, Kinney ME, Savik K, Gau JB, Wilcox C, Lerner I (2003) Therapeutic massage and healing touch improve symptoms in cancer. Integr Cancer Ther 2:332–344

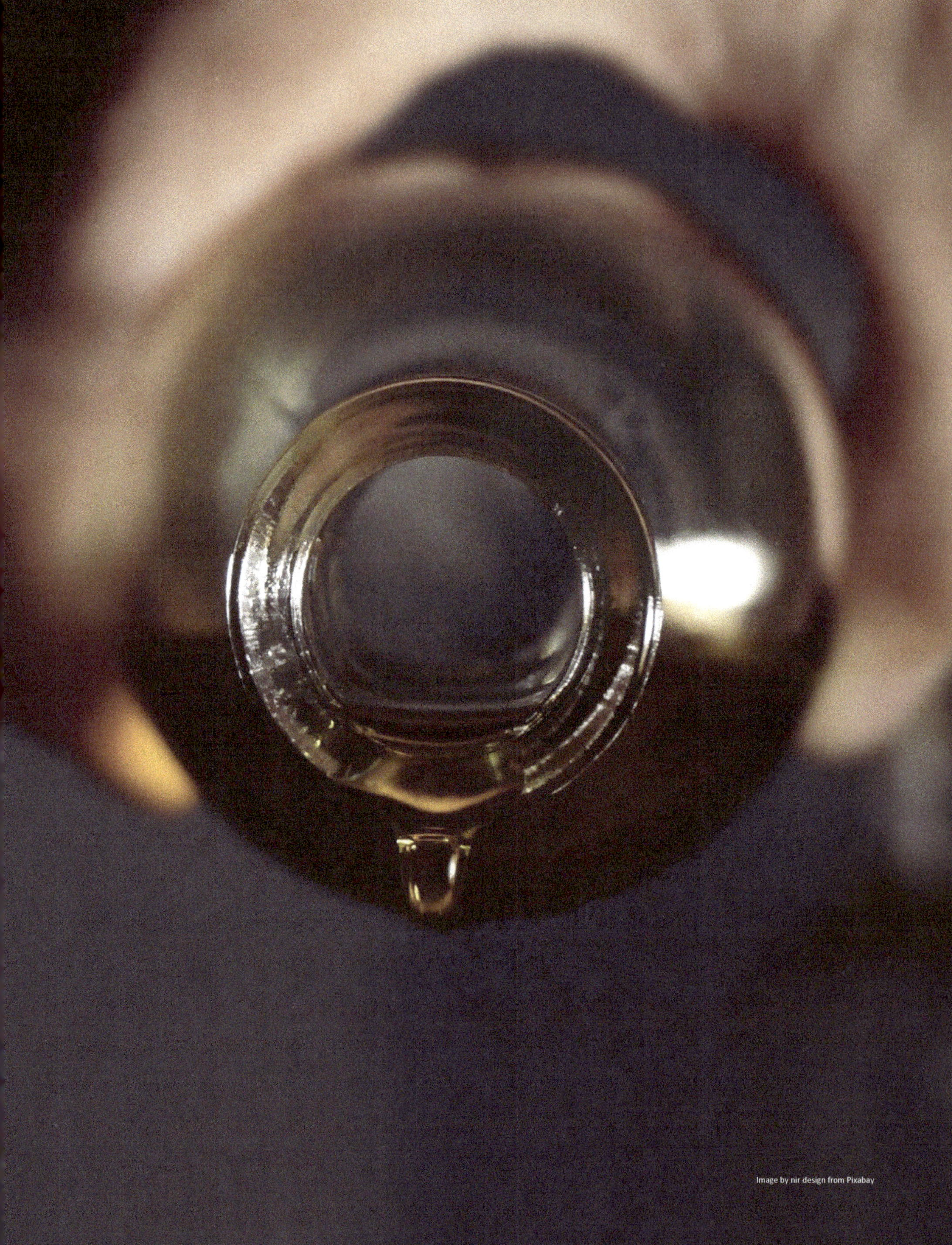

Image by nir design from Pixabay

Agarwood - Aquilaria crassna

Called the Scent of Heaven, the aromatic oil derived from the timber of this tree is considered to be the most beautiful aroma in the world. If you can afford this oil, then you are not depressed because you are poor, as it costs around US $50,000 per kilogram, which at the time I am writing this, is $8,000 more than pure gold per kilogram, making this tree one of the most valuable commodities in the world.

Agarwood is native to central Asia specifically Myanmar, Thailand, Vietnam, Laos, China, Bangladesh and the Philippines. There are approximately 31 species in the family with only 19 of them that produce the aromatic oil. The global demand and high prices for the timber are rapidly driving the species to extinction, however many new commercial plantations have also been established in the last decade or so. Traditionally the main markets for its 'oud oil' have been the Middle East, China, and Japan. Yet today it is sought after throughout the perfume industry. One drop of the oil in a well-known bottle of perfume may triple its price.

Throughout history there are references to the timber in various historical texts. It is referred to in the ancient Indian text Mahabharata which dates to the 1400 BCE. Also known as Aloe wood, a reference to the timber is found in the book of Numbers (24:6) in the Hebrew Bible. Ancient Greek writers also mention the tree and its uses. As a result, the trade in Agarwood started well before Christ came along and made Frankincense and Myrrh trendy. Buddha used Agarwood, and it is mentioned many times in the Buddhist texts, and in the Islam holy book, the Qur'an, there are multiple references to Aloe wood.

As can be imagined, due to the long history of use of Agarwood, there have been dozens of claims about its health attributes. The medicinal qualities that have been verified by science are the plant's anti-microbial, anti-inflammatory, laxative, anti-cancer, CNS depressant (helps with sleep and anxiety), analgesic and antidepressant qualities.

In research into the antidepressant actions of the oil, as well as the ethanol extract derived from the leaves, research found various chemical compounds that were responsible for the antidepressant actions, as well as a central nervous system depressant (relaxing) and anti-anxiety compounds. Compounds such as jinkoh-eremol, agarospirol from the extract, and benzylacetone, α-gurjunene, and (+)-calarene from the smoke vapour of the oil and wood, acted as a relaxant and increased sleep patterns. The presence of buagafuran has been associated with the antidepressant actions of Agarwood.

It is believed that buagafuran and similar compounds from Agarwood can positively affect the neurotransmitters such as dopamine. Additional research showed that Agarwood also had other significant compounds such as aquilarabietic acid A which showed remarkable antidepressant results in vivo. Along with these two compounds, a further 28 are currently being studied that are also believed to have antidepressant actions.

So, if you can afford this expensive oil of Agarwood called Oud, the research has shown it to have highly effective antidepressant qualities. Alternatively, if you live in the subtropical and tropical zones, the tree only takes fourteen years to make the oil. The wait might be worth its high profitably.

[1] S. Ahmed and S. Islam, "Aquilaria Crassna (Agarwood): Study of Pharmacological Activity and Medical Benefits," no. July, pp. 1–6, 2020.

[2] A. L. Sampson, "Growth physiology and productivity of cultivated Aquilaria cressna Pierre ex Lecomte (Thymelaeaceae) in tropical Australia and its reproduction biology," p. 139, 2017.

[3] S. Wang, Z. Yu, C. Wang, C. Wu, P. Guo, and J. Wei, "Chemical constituents and pharmacological activity of agarwood and aquilaria plants," Molecules, vol. 23, no. 2, 2018.

[4] S. Wang et al., "Agarwood essential oil ameliorates restrain stress-induced anxiety and depression by inhibiting HPA axis hyperactivity," Int. J. Mol. Sci., vol. 19, no. 11, 2018.

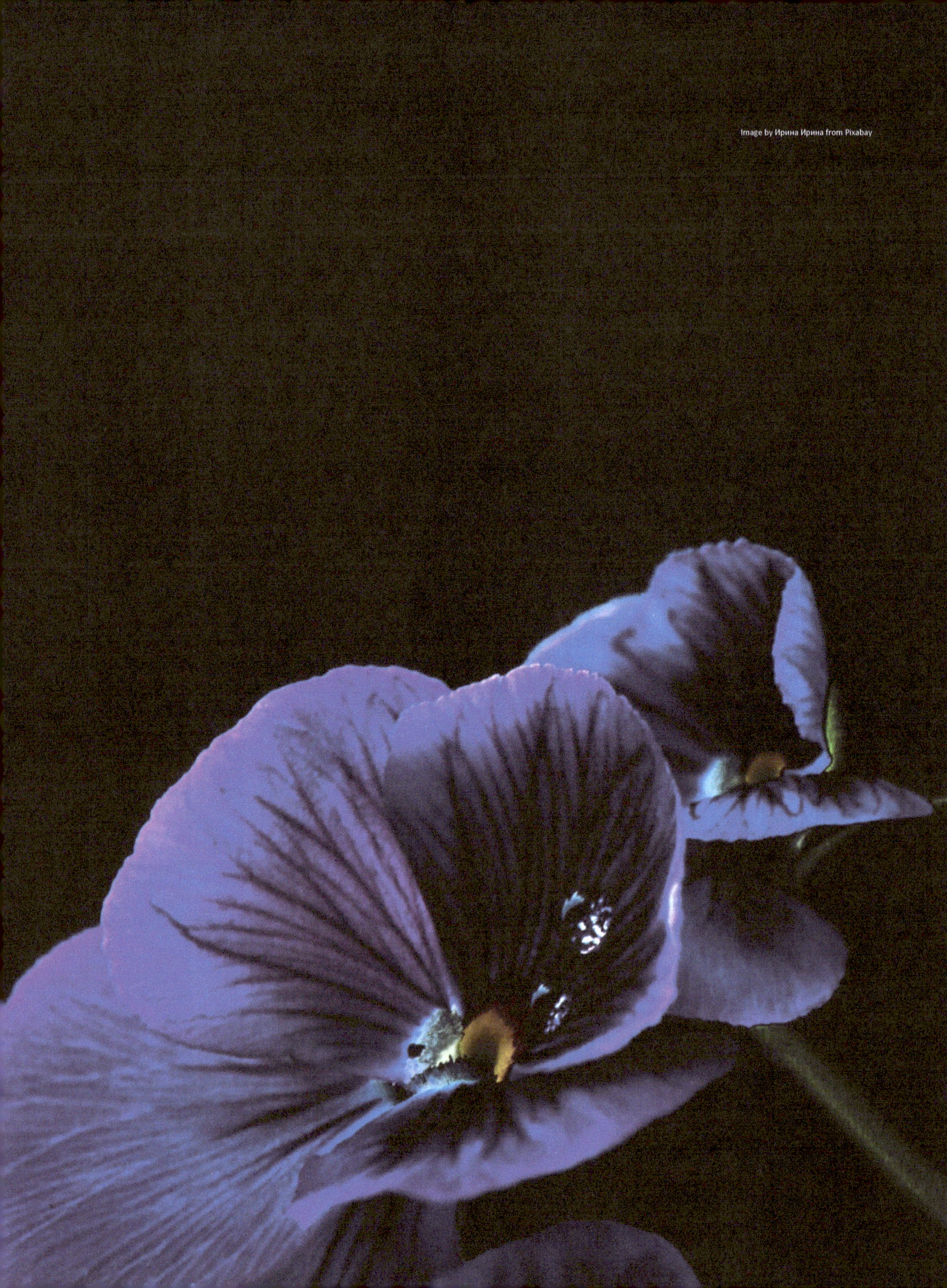
Image by Ирина Ирина from Pixabay

Sweet Violet - Viola odorata

This herb is part of a genus comprising more than 550 members, and is mainly found in the temperate Northern hemisphere, with a few of its members in Australia, South America and Hawaii. Violet odorata has a long history in Greek and Roman cultures and is associated with the Greek goddess of love and sexual pleasure, Aphrodite and her son Priapus. He lends his name to the medical condition known as Priapism or unusually large and permanent penile erections. The Romans were known to make a wine from the plant. This is intriguing as the herb is used to induce sleep, and therefore getting drunk with such a wine would be a very sleepy affair. The Romans, like the Greeks, associated the flower with the God Cupid, who was the god of love and desire. So, if someone gives you a bunch of flowers that are all Violets, they might be asking for something.

The predominant use of the plant is for the perfumery industry. The flowers and leaves have been used in medicine for thousands of years, and many ancient texts describe the use of the flower mainly for insomnia. The production of syrups and extracts has been reported to be diminishing in the last several decades.

In modern research, scientists have sought to understand the actions of the herb in the treatment of depression, anxiety and insomnia. In a paper from 2018, the herb was compared to various synthetic drugs, one of which was fluoxetine, and it found that its ethanol extract was comparable to it in the treatment of depression. Another paper from the same year corroborated the use of the plant for depression and highlighted doses ranging from 100 – 400 mg/kg body weight.

Viola odorata has been shown to be effective in reducing high blood pressure, comparable to the standard drug verapamil, and which is also used to treat migraine and cluster headaches. In doing so, Sweet Violet is thought to be a vasodilator and anti-inflammatory in action, and this explains its use in the treatment of bronchial asthma.

Whilst the herb is considered to be non-toxic, caution should be mentioned as the herb is also used as a laxative. So, should you decide to use the herb for your depression, you might also be detoxed and cleaned out, both mentally and physically.

[1] R. L. Delfanti et al., "No 主観的健康感を中心とした在宅高齢者における 健康関連指標に関する共分散構造分析Title," N. Engl. J. Med., vol. 372, no. 2, pp. 2499–2508, 2018.

[2] D. Chandra et al., "Phytochemical and Ethnomedicinal Uses of Family Violaceae," Curr. Res. Chem., vol. 7, no. 2, pp. 44–52, 2015.

[3] Z. Feyzabadi et al., "Efficacy of Viola odorata in treatment of chronic insomnia," Iran. Red Crescent Med. J., vol. 16, no. 12, 2014.

[4] N. Karim, I. Khan, A. Abdelhalim, A. Khan, and S. A. Halim, "Antidepressant potential of novel flavonoids derivatives from sweet violet (Viola odorata L): Pharmacological, biochemical and computational evidences for possible involvement of serotonergic mechanism," Fitoterapia, vol. 128, no. May, pp. 148–161, 2018.

[5] K. H. Janbaz, W. U. Khan, F. Saqib, and M. Khalid, "Pharmacological basis for the medicinal use of viola odorata in diarrhea, bronchial asthma and hypertension," Bangladesh J. Pharmacol., vol. 10, no. 4, pp. 836–843, 2015.

Depression is not sorry

"My recovery from depression has been an evolution, not a miracle!"

Patty Duke

As we have found out, the medical system and therapists around the world still struggle to find the cause or origin of depression. We hear words such as pathogenesis, meaning the manner of development of a disease, or aetiology, meaning the manner of causation of a disease or condition in the pursuit to solve depression's riddles and find a cure. Therefore, if our greatest medical minds are finding it hard to encapsulate depression, then it is no wonder that the internet is flooded with all manner of opinions and irresponsible claims concerning it. Yet, we know what it is not, which is sadness, self-pity, weakness or a choice.

The last one on our list is 'choice' which is pretty obvious, as no one ever said, "Hey I think today it would be cool to be depressed". Perhaps someone has feigned depression to get attention. This is a tool typically employed by those wielding 'self-pity' in an attempt to get what they want. Depression however has no goals or aims as it is devoid of the ego.

'Sadness' is a normal condition when we suffer loss. Loss of a loved one. Loss of a job. Loss of freedom. Loss of our dignity. However, sadness will eventually pass. Recovery is almost always assured. With this said, sadness if allowed to fester over a long time may result in depression, and with the original sadness forgotten in the end, it leaves only depression.

Imagine someone going about their daily life of work, family and social circles, all the time feeling worthless and empty. These people do not display 'weakness', they rather may be considered immensely strong as they battle their demons alone.

But perhaps the worst comparison or association of depression is to consider it to be a form of 'self-pity'. The simple act of feeling sorry for yourself is counter-intuitive in regard to depression as depression doesn't care. It just is. In most cases, a depressive person hides their depression. One of the challenges for therapists and friends is to actually get the person suffering from depression to actually talk about it. To open up to others is often extremely uncomfortable for several reasons, and the first of which is the expectation that other people will dismiss our fears as irrelevant. The second reason is that our fears may actually be validated by those around us, which makes our ugliness, inferiority, and worthlessness concrete. Yet in most cases, when a depressed person finally shares their fears, they are met with understanding even though the people listening to them cannot actually exactly know what is felt. Furthermore, the depressed person has one overriding fear, and that is that other people will actually pity them.

Self-pity is reserved for those people who blame the world, and everyone in it for their woes and lack. The simple statement "Why is this happening to me?" is the hallmark of self-pity, as it places the person in the centre of the question being afflicted by external negative events around them.

More often than not, a depressed person will think that they deserve the negatives that in some cases progress to an all-pervading numbness that simply is.

Self-pity, in most cases, can easily be solved if the person wants to. This 'if' is a big IF, as the everyday self-pitying advocate is seeking attention and help from others, because they have the opinion that they deserve as much, and possibly more. They have placed their happiness at the control of external things and people. They want an apology from someone who has done them wrong. They want people to demonstrate their desire for them. They want to be recognised. In short, they want a lot. And all of it is external to themselves. Therefore, as long as they externalise their causes, they are actually making themselves powerless to change as they await in futility for the world to recognize them and apologise. The world really doesn't care. Never has and never will! So, these people in the self-pity camp are pretty miserable, but definitely not depressed. Insecure most definitely. Yet, what must be done is to finally accept that no apology is coming. No accolades, and no one else is going to bring them eternal happiness. They simply need to accept that they are the creators of their own present reality, even if other people have been mean or unkind to them. Once they do this, then they take back control from others and will be able to move forwards.

Depression is not sorry. For it to be that it would have to be a thing. Something, an action, a cause, a condition, a tool. Depression is not sorry, because it is a 'nothing' into which good people disappear.

Dogs know nothing of self-pity as they have already given you everything.

[1] de Souza, L.K., Policarpo, D. & Hutz, C.S. Self-compassion and Symptoms of Stress, Anxiety, and Depression. Trends in Psychol. 28, 85–98 (2020). https://doi.org/10.1007/s43076-020-00018-2

[2] https://drmargaretrutherford.com/is-it-self-pity-depression-or-perfectly-hidden-depression/

[3] K. M. Douglas and R. M. Sutton, "Kent Academic Repository," Eur. J. Soc. Psychol., vol. 40, no. 2, pp. 366–374, 2010.

[4] J. Stöber, "Self-Pity: Exploring the Links to Personality, Control Beliefs, and Anger," J. Pers., vol. 71, no. 2, pp. 183–220, 2003.

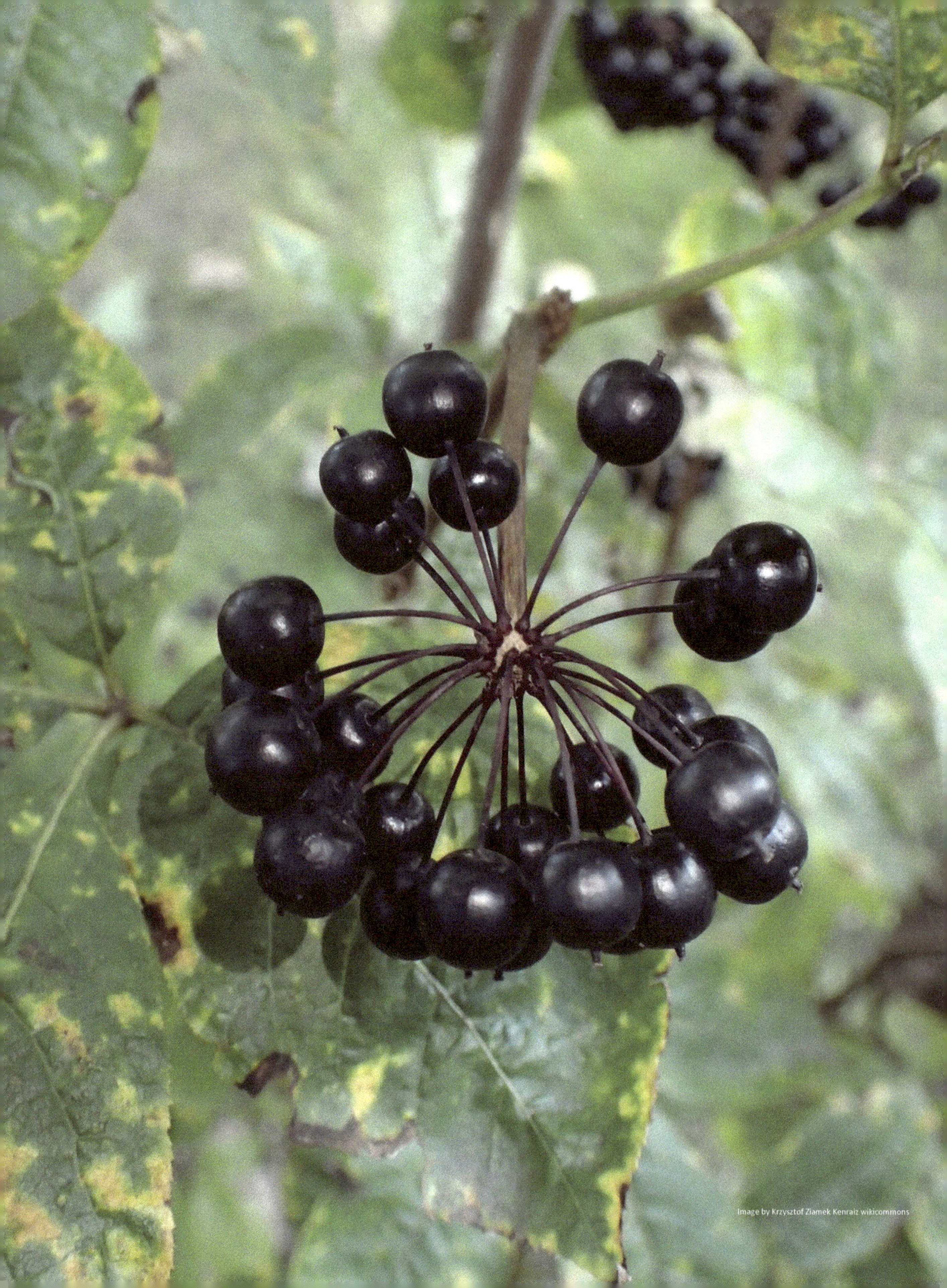

Image by Krzysztof Ziamek Kenraiz wikicommons

Siberian Ginseng - Eleutherococus senticosus

This herb comes from the Taiga region of Siberia, hence the name. It is also found in Northern China and Japan. The indigenous people from these regions have long used the herb, and references to it date back almost 2000 years. There is some confusion around it as the plant has two or more different scientific names, one being Acanthopanax senticosus. Yet the common names are Siberian Ginseng, Devils Bush, Shigoka and more recently merely Eleuthro. In America it cannot be sold as Siberian Ginseng as this was successfully challenged by the growers and manufacturers of the authentic Ginseng (Panax). Therefore, it is now illegal to sell the herb using the term ginseng in that region of the world.

In Chinese medicine, eleuthero is used as a powerful tonic which we know as an adaptogen. Basically, an adaptogen is an herbal drug that has an overall strengthening of the entire body with particular emphasis on reducing stress. When reviewing eleuthero, it has been found to be beneficial to several of the body's systems such as cardiac, pulmonary, liver, renal and skeletal systems. Concerning the plants' ability to reduce symptoms of depression, various studies have been undertaken. They have resulted in a large body of scientific evidence of the plants' support for the central nervous system (CNS). Studies from 2009 and 2010 showed that the significant support for the CNS and especially brain tissue resulted from a dose of 100 mg/kg in mice. It is thought that the compound unique to eleuthro, known as eleutheroside B, was responsible and significantly reduced inflammation in brain tissue.

More specific research from 2013 showed that the aqueous extract from the plant significantly up-regulated (increased) norepinephrine as well as dopamine levels in mice, thereby reducing depression. However, the doses used in this study from China were quite large at 2000 mg/kg body weight. The good news is that a simple tisane made from the leaves or fruits from the plant will be effective, albeit several cups will be needed. Traditionally the roots are the part of the plant most used in making extracts, yet the stems contain higher levels of eleutherosides, indicating that the whole plant may be used.

In these studies, it was found that whilst Siberian ginseng was effective in CNS support and cognitive function, it was not as effective as imipramine in the management of depression. Regardless, it had significant positive effects on concentration and learning.

Other positive effects found from the use of Siberian ginseng is the reduction in fatigue or to put it the other way, an increase in energy. Also, the extract showed significant protection against ulcerative conditions of the bowel. In all, it is reported that there are more than 1,000 articles on this plant, and it is in use all over the world.

[1] L. Z. Huang, H. F. Zhao, B. K. Huang, C. J. Zheng, W. Peng, and L. P. Qin, "Acanthopanax senticosus: Review of botany, chemistry and pharmacology," Pharmazie, vol. 66, no. 2, pp. 83–97, 2011.

[2] X. Wang, Y. Zhang, and T. Chinese, "Eleutherococcus senticosus Systematic Characterization of the Absorbed Components of Acanthopanax senticosus Stem How to use the monographs Rapid Analysis of Constituents and Metabolites From Extracts of Acanthopanax senticosus Harms Leaf," 2017.

[3] N. Asia et al., "Eleutherococcus senticosus," pp. 4–6.

[4] B. Muszyńska, M. Łojewski, J. Rojowski, W. Opoka, and K. Sułkowska-Ziaja, "Natural products of relevance in the prevention and supportive treatment of depression," Psychiatr. Pol., vol. 49, no. 3, pp. 435–453, 2015.

[5] European Medicines Agency, "Assessment report on Eleutherococcus senticosus," Eur. Med. Agency, vol. 44, no. May, 2014.

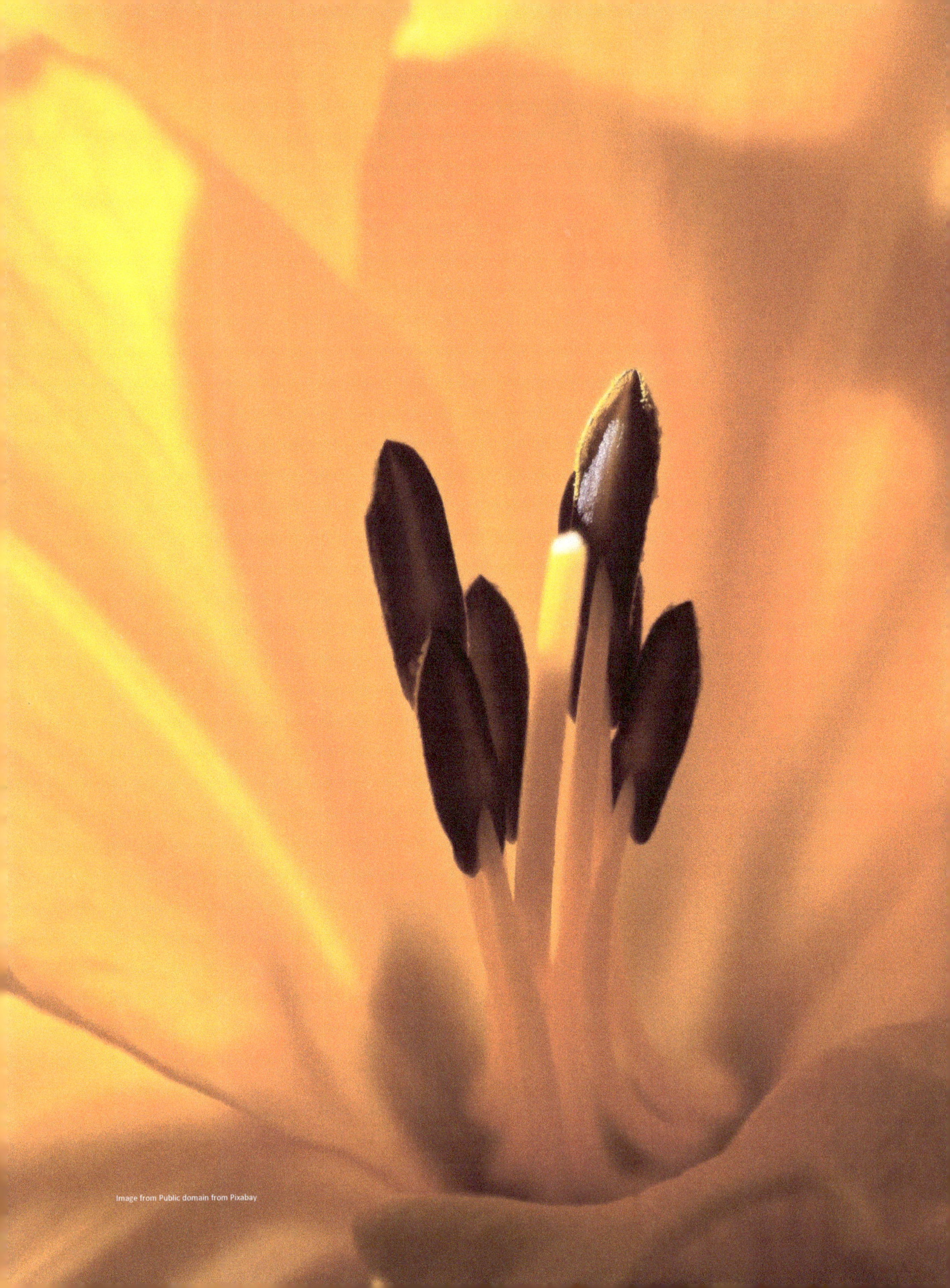

Image from Public domain from Pixabay

Daylily - Hemerocallis citrina

Daylily is native to East Asia and China and is predominantly used as a vegetable in the cuisines of several countries there. The dried petals of the flowers are added to soups, curries, and other dishes to impart colour and flavour. In addition to the daily use of the plant as a food, it has been utilised for centuries as an essential medicine, and one of its common names in China is wang yu cao, roughly translated as "forget-one's sadness".

Recent research has concentrated on the ethanol extract of the flowers and it has resulted in wide ranging support for the use of the plant in the management of depression.

A systematic review of scientific research into the efficacy of Hemerocallis was published in Poland in 2019 and compiled a library of over 290 research papers profiling both Hemerocallis and Gladioli concerning the antidepressant activity of both plants. The findings from the review showed that the primary actions of Hemerocallis were its anti-inflammatory and antioxidant benefits. The researchers also believed that the high levels of both rutin and hesperidin contributed to its beneficial effects. Other actions of Daylily indicated that the ethanol extract inhibited the reuptake of the monoamine neurotransmitters dopamine, noradrenaline and serotonin.

An earlier paper from 2014, published in China, found that a dosage of 400 mg/kg of ethanol flower extract exhibited significant antidepressant actions. The researchers went one step further and also tested their hypothesis by using only rutin and hesperidin and found that these two compounds had the same effect in the alleviation of depressive symptoms. Within this scientific study it found that the plant is nontoxic, and at doses of 5000 mg/kg no adverse effects were noted.

Another study also from China (2017) sought to further test the claim that rutin and hesperidin were the sole compounds responsible for the actions of Daylily. In this research the scientists hypothesised that other compounds found within the plant may also contribute to antidepressant actions. Whilst both rutin and hesperidin are flavonoids, the authors of this 2017 study postulated that phenols may also contribute. To this end, they isolated factions of the plant extract and found that whilst rutin and hesperidin did indeed increase levels of precursors for serotonin, they also increased acetylcholinesterase. It was the phenolic acids of the plant that directly influenced the level of dopamine. As a conclusion we can see the complex nature of plant extracts and the symphony of organic chemistry that cautions against the desire to focus on merely one unique compound, but rather utilise the whole plant extract.

[1] B. Du et al., "Antidepressant-like effects of the hydroalcoholic extracts of Hemerocallis Citrina and its potential active components," BMC Complement. Altern. Med., vol. 14, no. 1, pp. 1–11, 2014.

[2] K. Solati, M. Asadi-Samani, and S. Heidari-Soureshjani, "Medicinal Plants Effective on Serotonin Level: A Systematic Review," J. Pharm. Res. Int., vol. 19, no. 4, pp. 1–12, 2017.

[3] D. Distribution et al., "Hemerocallis citrina," no. January 2016, pp. 19–20, 2020.

[4] R. Matraszek-Gawron, M. Chwil, P. Terlecka, and M. M. Skoczylas, "Recent studies on anti-depressant bioactive substances in selected species from the genera hemerocallis and gladiolus: A systematic review," Pharmaceuticals, vol. 12, no. 4, 2019.

[5] H. Tian et al., "Effects of phenolic constituents of daylily flowers on corticosterone- and glutamate-treated PC12 cells," BMC Complement. Altern. Med., vol. 17, no. 1, pp. 1–12, 2017.

The hidden pollution

"You don't drown by falling in water, you drown by staying there!"

Edwin Louis Cole

If you like conspiracy theories, then you are going to love this section. And if you love science then you may like it even more so! We have discussed the global trend where depression is becoming the fourth leading contributor to the global burden of disease. And this trend is not slowing down as it is expected to become the second leading cause in the coming decade. Around the world, health researchers are seeking to understand more about depression whilst also seeking cures. When we analyse global trends that are common to all societies, we can find correlations in diet, employment, exercise, and technology. One such correlation between depression can be found in the telecommunications and computing industries, where more and more people are living in a connected world, requiring people to swim in a hidden sea of energy networks. Is this growth in technology a possible mirror of the growth of depression?

The debate around the health risks of wireless technologies has emerged from the previous debates around electromagnetic radiation (EMR) from high voltage power lines in the late 1980's and 90's. The debate rages onward and whilst the science exposing the risk becomes more voluminous, counterclaims continue. I simply take the view of Gain versus Loss. Is there a party with a risk as to the outcome of the debate proving harm? The answer is "of course there is!". The parties with the most to lose are the telecommunication industry and the governments that are aware of the societal and economic impacts should the health risks become endorsed. Against this are the researchers who have little to gain and much to lose as reputations are put at stake. Therefore, it may be that another industry is denying their products are unsafe in much the same manner as we have seen in the tobacco industry, and the fossil fuel industries. Herein lies the 'conspiracy theory' paradigm. In this section we will start at one extreme and travel to the opposing extreme, to hopefully arrive at a middle ground where a balanced educated assessment is produced.

Ask the question "Can harm to a person occur from electromagnetic radiation, microwaves and/or radio waves?". The best place to start reviewing this statement is with the military. In the war rooms of the world, no one continues to talk about laser technology in isolation any more, they talk about directed energy weapons (DEW), because the application of not simply lasers (light) but also radio (RF), microwave (MW) and electromagnetic (EMF) are now mainstream. If any of this is true, which we have no doubt that it is, then the effects of such radiation and or energy weapons are of interest, and the funding continues to flow into the research into them. The discussions about DEW are well crafted as the accepted context is to talk of 'defensive' applications, and an aggressive enemy may be disrupted or stopped via the use of DEW that interrupt communications, computers (aircraft, navy etc.) and transport. Yet the research into the use of DEW to inflict harm on enemy soldiers or worse, a nation's own citizens, is less transparent. Therefore, the labels 'non-lethal' and 'lethal' have had to be used for DEW and in doing so, we have a truly clear understanding that there is a risk of harm and even death from radio frequency, microwave and electromagnetic fields. The differentiation between lethal DEW and non-lethal DEW was highlighted in the TECOM Technology Symposium, as far back as 1997, where it was stated that one of the limiting factors in testing such weapons were the people themselves, because the possible permanent damage to test subjects was far too great.

It is thought that the incident at the US Embassy in Havana Cuba in 2016 was indeed an attack on the diplomats, staff, and families, by DEW's. Within the official reports on the event, where the people inside the embassy suffered from cognitive function, sleep disorders, headaches and hearing mysterious sounds, it is stated that the cause is unknown. And various highly regarded scientists publicly stated that the symptoms were almost identical to those in Japan by people who suffered from electromagnetic radiation. Once again, in 2018, a similar event occurred in Guangzhou China, also on American staff who had to be evacuated and treated in the States. The coincidence is far too disturbing for it to be either random or of natural causes.

As can be seen in this example, it is possible to weaponize the same energies that are in our microwaves, sound systems and wireless routers. To say without hesitation that heating, communication, and sounds pose no threat is puerile at best. Dramatic impacts on health have been well established at musical events where the sound levels exceed a normal range. If music can hurt us, then it may be feasible that any other form of vibrational energy has an equal or greater chance of doing so as well. Yet, before we launch into pseudo-science and surrender ourselves to irrational arguments, it becomes apparent that we have to first understand the question, or even more important find the right question as our starting point.

The counterclaim is that the frequency levels required to cause harm need to be of such a high magnitude that the prevailing or current levels within our societies are so low that they can pose no direct influence on our health. However, this is a facile argument, and it is similarly used in the discussion on pharmaceutical drugs. With a chemical cure, a drug at low levels may have no health benefit whatsoever, therefore the correct dosage is essential. An excessive dose on the other hand may have detrimental or fatal results. Hence a beneficial medicine ceases to be a cure and becomes a poison. Actually, no one is arguing against the correct dosage and known benefit. Electromagnetic radiation (ER) is now being researched as a tool in a possible health cure scenario. Therefore, one can agree that it has an effect on our bodies. This makes the claims that EMF, RF and MW pose no adverse effect on society's health are 'null and void'. It either has an effect or it has not. The current field of research into this topic universally agrees that it has an effect. The debate is about whether the effect is negative or benign.

The human body is a complex biological 'receiver' for all manner of energy. We can be thought of as soft mechanical and chemical machines that employ both chemical and electrical communications networks internally. It has been shown that the human body actually reacts in the same manner as a 'capacitor', a fancy name for a battery. We can store energy, and we can also lose energy. Accordingly, we are receptive to external stimuli. One of the most common stimuli is sunlight on which we are dependent upon for all life itself. The childhood medical condition known as Ricketts is where the bones and teeth become soft and deformed due to Vitamin D deficiency. Therapy for this malady was to sit children in sunlight well before we truly understood the association between ultraviolet B radiation and vitamin D synthesis. These children in the 1920's as an image, all lined up in a row sitting in full sunlight, bring us to the first extreme. If you thought it was the military at the other extreme, then you were wrong. The petty and vacuous striving of generals and politicians for power and wealth is of an insignificant level of stupidity when we think of the sun.

This life-giving orb we and other planets hug for dear life is especially pertinent for our little earth and the microbes living on it, us. The sun is a gargantuan burning ball of plasma emitting a vast amount of energy in the form of ultraviolet, basic light, heat, radio waves and a raft of other types of radiation that washes over us daily. Yet at times our sun develops a slight wobble and may release what is known as a solar flare. One of these solar flares hit Canada head on in August 1989. This discharge of enormous amounts of solar radiation caused the main Quebec power station to go off-line, creating a power outage or black-out for 9 hours. The wave of energy overpowered the high-voltage power lines of the electricity grid and plunged the nation into darkness. This is an extreme example of basic electrical engineering where a large more powerful electromagnetic field influences and negatively disrupts a lesser current. Therefore, consider the immense energy being emitted by the sun every moment, and compare this to one of the neurons in the average person's brain that has been measured as giving off between -80 to -40 microvolts when active. The neurons that allow us to think, remember, talk, walk, and basically function, are the other extreme in this discussion.

It is estimated that the sun delivers approximately 120 watts of power to every square meter of ground on earth. When compared to the estimated power output of the average human body of 100 Watts at any given time, we can feel relatively calm about our natural environment because the disparity is small. The human species along with every other species on this planet evolved under these conditions and have adapted accordingly. The environment on our beloved Terra Firma has always been a soup of water, air, chemicals, temperatures, natural forces and also electromagnetic radiations. We have been shaped by all of these influences, and to say one has had little impact would be a hard position to defend scientifically. Needless to say, in recent centuries, we humans have altered the natural environment drastically to a point where our influence on the natural order is anything but 'normal'. This is the case when it comes to our use of energy technologies such as electricity, wireless, microwave and radio frequencies. Earth has always possessed vast amounts of carbon dioxide, and yet our influence on the levels of this simple compound of a 'carbon molecule linking two oxygen molecules' may well kill us all. It is the same with electromagnetic radiation.

Much of the research prior to 2000 into the possible health risks of energy systems focused on cancer and its prevalence near power grids. Until recently the research did not seek to understand the more subtle effects these frequencies had on other bodily systems such as the central nervous system and brain function. Over the past decade and longer, scientists and researchers have become more vocal on health impacts from EMF technologies that are emerging at an ever-faster rate.

It has been found in research that an extremely low-frequency electromagnetic field (ELF-EMF) has a disruptive action on the replication of DNA in the human body. This research from Romania was published in 2015 and questioned the claims that ELF-EMF fields were safe. Their findings disputed such claims, and even went so far as to warn against exposure, stating that "ELF-EMF of 100 Hz and 5.6 mT had a genotoxic impact on Vero cells." In short, the ELF-EMF caused damage to the genetic information within cells, and this in turn caused mutations that may be a precursor for various cancers. The low frequency of 100 Hz was chosen by the researchers as this level is common in electric cars, trains, and medical devices. A paper from India in 2013 hypothesised that both low and high frequency EMF enhanced the chance of autism in children due to the damage to the gene coding of the body. Moving outward from DNA and arriving at the cellular level, we have known that every cell in the human body generates small amounts of electricity in order to carry out various chemical processes and functions. In the muscle cells and neurons of the central nervous system, the cells not only use electricity to function but also to communicate. Every cell has what is known as 'membrane potential', and this is the difference between the interior and exterior charge or potential. Covering a cell wall are the various 'ion gates' that allow sodium, potassium, chloride and calcium to pass through. The potassium gate is the most abundant and complex and requires 100 genes for function. Now let's go further out and see the entire human body.

This wondrous machine that uses mechanical (muscles and bones) and chemical (basically everything from food to brain function) and then onto energy (both thermal and electrical) we finally come to the skin. This outer membrane keeps us all in one piece. The skin acts not only as a barrier against our bacterial and viral environments, but it also helps to regulate fluids, oxygen and also electricity. It has been shown that an external current is mediated by the skin. It acts as an insulator. When the skin is broken or bypassed (orally) the current flows freely. An electrical shock that passed through the skin is moderated. However, if the current is large enough it can blow a hole through this outer barrier that we all take for granted, causing unrivalled havoc on our biology. This is why, when you hold a 9-volt square battery to your skin you will feel nothing. However, place the poles on your tongue and you have a whole different matter. It will shock you. We humans are a marvellous creation, and part of this creation is its ability to make and store electricity.

It has been found that a Low Frequency Magnetic field will stimulate the body's immune system by activating the cytokine response critical for the modulation of the immune system. Research in some areas seek to understand this response from an EMF in much more detail, and hopefully employ it in disease control, with perhaps a role in cancer prevention and management. Other research has shown however that this cytokine response elicited within the body by an EMF may potentially cause autoimmune disease and the inflammatory response that accompanies it. As we know, inflammation is closely associated with depression. This then leads us into EMFs and their role in psychosomatic conditions of which depression is one.

We will talk about suicide in more detail later when we consider that depression affects potentially one in four people globally. In the United States however, suicide is the eighth largest cause of death. So why then has research focused on electricity grids and a possible association with suicide, as was presented in a report from 2000 that was funded by the Electric Power Research Institute of Palo Alto, California, and carried out by a team of scientists from the university of North Carolina. The findings from this research paper presented enough data to see a link between an increase in suicide rates in its line workers, the men and women who daily work directly with power grids, that was unlike their counterparts who worked in management, administration, maintenance, or positions that did not bring the person into exposure to the EMF radiation. The conclusion from this report states that "The results of this study provide evidence for an association between cumulative exposure of extremely low– frequency EMFs and suicide, especially among younger workers. We hypothesise that an increased vulnerability at younger ages may be based on a change in the nature of depression with age, with suicide more closely linked to depression among younger workers and physical impairments among older workers". While the report sent out a warning about ELF-EMF, it was the focus on the age of the affected group from the 138,905 men included in the report. In more and more reports, it was found that the younger generations are more susceptible to EMF induced psychosomatic problems.

An abundance of research is being written on the effects extremely low frequency EMFs are having on our bodies. Yet, perhaps the strongest evidence is the effect they are having on the immune system in our bodies. Research from Italy, The Netherlands, Sweden, Austria and others all showed that ELF-EMF does disrupt the body's immune system. This in turn creates support for other research into the inflammatory response alone created by ELF-EMF. Research from 2014 states; "Furthermore, appropriate exposure assessment is crucial for the identification of dose-response relation if any, and the elucidation of the biological interaction mechanism. For the time being, the public should follow the precautionary principle and limit their exposure as much as possible". In 2017, other research supported the claims of papers such as the 2014 paper and others, but it also showed that the ELF-EMF also reduced antioxidants' ability to work effectively. An analogy for this would be alike seeing a fire and all the fire extinguishers were empty. Antioxidants, as their title implies, reduce oxidation in the tissues of the body, reduce inflammatory conditions. So, not only does EMF stimulate the immune system resulting in inflammation, but the EMF also negates our beneficial regulatory response by restricting the actions of antioxidants.

The medical treatments for depression focus on the monoamine neurotransmitters via the use of reuptake inhibitors and other medications. Yet, an underlying process known as Voltage Regulated Calcium Channel Activation is a primary trigger for the release of these neurotransmitters and neuroendocrine hormones. Two studies from 2015, one from Shanghai University and the other from Washington State University, discuss the effect that LF-EMF has on this calcium exchange on the cellular level across the entire neuronal network of the central nervous system. Whilst the Chinese study purely looked at the chemical interactions of the calcium exchange and the influence the EMF had on the process, the paper from Washington State University, written by Mr Martin L. Pall Professor Emeritus of Biochemistry and Basic Medical Science, discussed the neuropsychiatric effects. Professor Paal cites over 80 studies, and his paper is actually a meta-analysis of research over 50 years. He concluded with the following statement: "With ever-increasing exposures in human populations, we have no idea what the consequences of these ever-increasing exposures will be". He lists the following neuropsychiatric conditions caused by Low Level EMF as sleep disturbance / insomnia, headache, fatigue / tiredness, dysesthesia, concentration / attention dysfunction, memory changes, dizziness, irritability, loss of appetite / body weight, restlessness / anxiety, nausea, skin burning / tingling / dermographism, EEG changes and depression / depressive symptoms.

We could go on discussing numerous studies and papers, yet this would be tiresome and pointless as the basic premise has been portrayed, which is that "the human body is able to generate electricity on a cellular level, which is essential for the basic functioning of our biology. The evidence is clear that other electromagnetic fields, frequencies and radiation will of course interact with the body's chemistry resulting in both positive and negative outcomes. However, the negative repercussions are by far the most common".

Here we are now surrounded by this invisible pollution, and it has the potential to induce depression. So, what can be done to protect ourselves in this new world order? Obviously reducing our exposure to these EMFs would be the most obvious. Wherever possible, distance yourself from your mobile cellular phones. It is recommended to either turn them off when you sleep, or place them at least four meters away from the bed and possibly in another room altogether. Turn off the Wi-Fi at night. A good way of doing this is to connect the Wi-Fi router to a timer switch whereby it automatically turns off at a predetermined time and then on again in the morning. You can also purchase specially designed mobile phone cases that inhibit radiation exposure. Furthermore, ascertain where the wiring is in your home and position the furniture accordingly, especially your bed.

In recent years, an activity known as 'forest bathing' has increased in popularity. Immersing yourself in forests and rural settings where there are no power lines or mobile networks has been adopted by many people as a method of rebalancing the body and eliciting feelings of well-being. A unique and now obvious therapy was developed first in Germany in the 1920s and then more formally in the manner of assisted (equipment) in the late 20th century in America known as 'grounding' or 'earthing'. The basic premise is that the body has the potential to act as a 'capacitor' (a battery), for it can store excess electrical energy. And, simply connecting the body to the ground/earth, either by walking barefoot or attaching a copper cable to the body via clothing or bed sheets, can release this excess energy into the ground. Like all modalities, there will be those who believe and those who do not. This therapy is no different and has various nay-sayers who ridicule the practice. However, the anti-earthing activists, whilst having the best of intentions, are largely employing simplistic arguments of electrical engineering, such as shoes are not good insulators and therefore the body is continually discharging even when we wear shoes. Yet, this is entirely dependent on the voltage being discussed, and in the human body the electrical capacity is not large enough to 'jump' through the most basic insulation. An extreme example of this can be seen in the case studies of people struck by lightning. A great deal of these victims had their shoes blown off their feet as the voltage contained in the lightning is so strong their shoes offer no protection whatsoever.

Further, we have discussed the evolutionary environment in which we and all other life have developed on earth within an electromagnetic soup created by the relationship between the sun and the earth. This creation has been radically changed in the past few hundred years by the development of technologies to a point where this electromagnetic environment is significantly more active than its original baseline. We learned that a very small amount of electromagnetic field interference is all we need on our bodies for the cellular activity to be disruptive.

As a result, a method to reduce this would clearly be beneficial. Therefore, the simple act of walking barefoot on moist soil may well be the thing you need to lift your spirits. Instinctively your dog will follow and sense the serenity.

[1] M. Ryan, M. R. Frater, and M. J. Ryan, 'The Impact of Radio Frequency Directed Energy Weapons (RF DEW) on the Modern Battlefield Managing Uncertainties and Disruptions in Project Scheduling View project INCOSE Requirements Working Group View project The Impact of Radio-Frequency Directed Energy,' no. January, 2000.

[2] R. Watson-watt, 'Directed-energy weapon,' 2019.

[3] T. Fritze, S. Teipel, A. Óvári, I. Kilimann, G. Witt, and G. Doblhammer, 'Hearing Impairment Affects Dementia Incidence. An Analysis Based on Longitudinal Health Claims Data in Germany,' PLoS One, vol. 11, no. 7, p. e0156876, 2016.

[4] M. L. Pall, 'Microwave frequency electromagnetic fields (EMFs) produce widespread neuropsychiatric effects including depression,' Journal of Chemical Neuroanatomy, vol. 75. pp. 43–51, 2016.

[5] W. Edwin and C. Image, 'The hidden pollution.' 2001.

[6] F. Church, 'Cellular Phone,' SpringerReference, 2011.

[7] P. Boscolo, M. Di Gioacchino, L. Di Giampaolo, A. Antonucci, and S. Di Luzio, 'Combined effects of electromagnetic fields on immune and nervous responses.,' Int. J. Immunopathol. Pharmacol., vol. 20, no. 2 Suppl 2, pp. 59–63, 2007.

[8] J. R. Hoehn, 'Defence Primer : Military Use of the Electromagnetic Spectrum,' 2019.

[9] 'A review on the effects of extremely low frequency electromagnetic field.' .

[10] S. Singh and N. Kapoor, 'Health Implications of Electromagnetic Fields, Mechanisms of Action, and Research Needs,' Adv. Biol., vol. 2014, pp. 1–24, 2014.

[11] O. Johansson, 'Disturbance of the immune system by electromagnetic fields-A potentially underlying cause for cellular damage and tissue repair reduction which could lead to disease and impairment,' Pathophysiology, vol. 16, no. 2–3, pp. 157–177, 2009.

[12] 'inflammation.' .

[13] M. M. Rosado, M. Simkó, M.-O. Mattsson, and C. Pioli, 'Immune-Modulating Perspectives for Low Frequency Electromagnetic Fields in Innate Immunity,' Front. Public Heal., vol. 6, no. March, pp. 1–13, 2018.

[14] G. Redlarski et al., 'The influence of electromagnetic pollution on living organisms: Historical trends and forecasting changes,' Biomed Res. Int., vol. 2015, 2015.

[15] M. Reale and P. Amerio, 'Extremely low frequency electromagnetic field and cytokines production,' Electromagnetic Fields: Principles, Engineering Applications and Biophysical Effects. pp. 239–253, 2013.

[16] L. A. Golbach, M. H. Scheer, J. J. M. Cuppen, H. Savelkoul, and B. M. L. Verburg-Van Kemenade, 'Low-Frequency Electromagnetic Field Exposure Enhances Extracellular Trap Formation by Human Neutrophils through the NADPH Pathway,' J. Innate Immun., vol. 7, no. 5, pp. 459–465, 2015.

[17] M. L. Pall, 'Microwave frequency electromagnetic fields (EMFs) produce widespread neuropsychiatric effects including depression,' J. Chem. Neuroanat., vol. 75, no. August, pp. 43–51, 2016.

[18] Y. R. Ahuja, S. Sharma, and B. Bahadur, 'Autism: An epigenomic side-effect of excessive exposure to electromagnetic fields,' Int. J. Med. Med. Sci., vol. 5, no. 4, pp. 171–177, 2013.

[19] B. B. Levitt and H. Lai, 'Biological effects from exposure to electromagnetic radiation emitted by cell tower base stations and other antenna arrays,' Environ. Rev., vol. 18, no. 1, pp. 369–395, 2010.
[20] G. Chevalier, S. T. Sinatra, J. L. Oschman, K. Sokal, and P. Sokal, 'Earthing: Health implications of reconnecting the human body to the Earth's surface electrons,' J. Environ. Public Health, vol. 2012, 2012.
[21] 'Disturbance of the immune system by electromagnetic fields—A potentially underlying cause for cellul.'.
[22] A. Višnjić et al., 'Relationship between the manner of mobile phone use and depression, anxiety, and stress in university students,' Int. J. Environ. Res. Public Health, vol. 15, no. 4, pp. 1–11, 2018.
[23] E. Van Wijngaarden, D. A. Savitz, R. C. Kleckner, J. Cai, and D. Loomis, 'Exposure to electromagnetic fields and suicide among electric utility workers: A nested case-control study,' Occup. Environ. Med., vol. 57, no. 4, pp. 258–263, 2000.
[24] J. E. Keller-Byrne and F. Akbar-Khanzadeh, 'Potential emotional and cognitive disorders associated with exposure to EMFs: A Review,' AAOHN J., vol. 45, no. 2, pp. 69–75, 1997.
[25] 'Diplomats' mystery illness linked to radiofrequency microwave radiation, researcher says -- ScienceDaily.'.
[26] M. F. Holick, 'Sunlight and vitamin D for bone health and prevention of autoimmune diseases, cancers, and cardiovascular disease.,' Am. J. Clin. Nutr., vol. 80, no. 6 Suppl, pp. 1678–1688, 2004.
[27] C. H. Lee and F. Giuliani, 'The Role of Inflammation in Depression and Fatigue,' Front. Immunol., vol. 10, no. July, p. 1696, 2019.

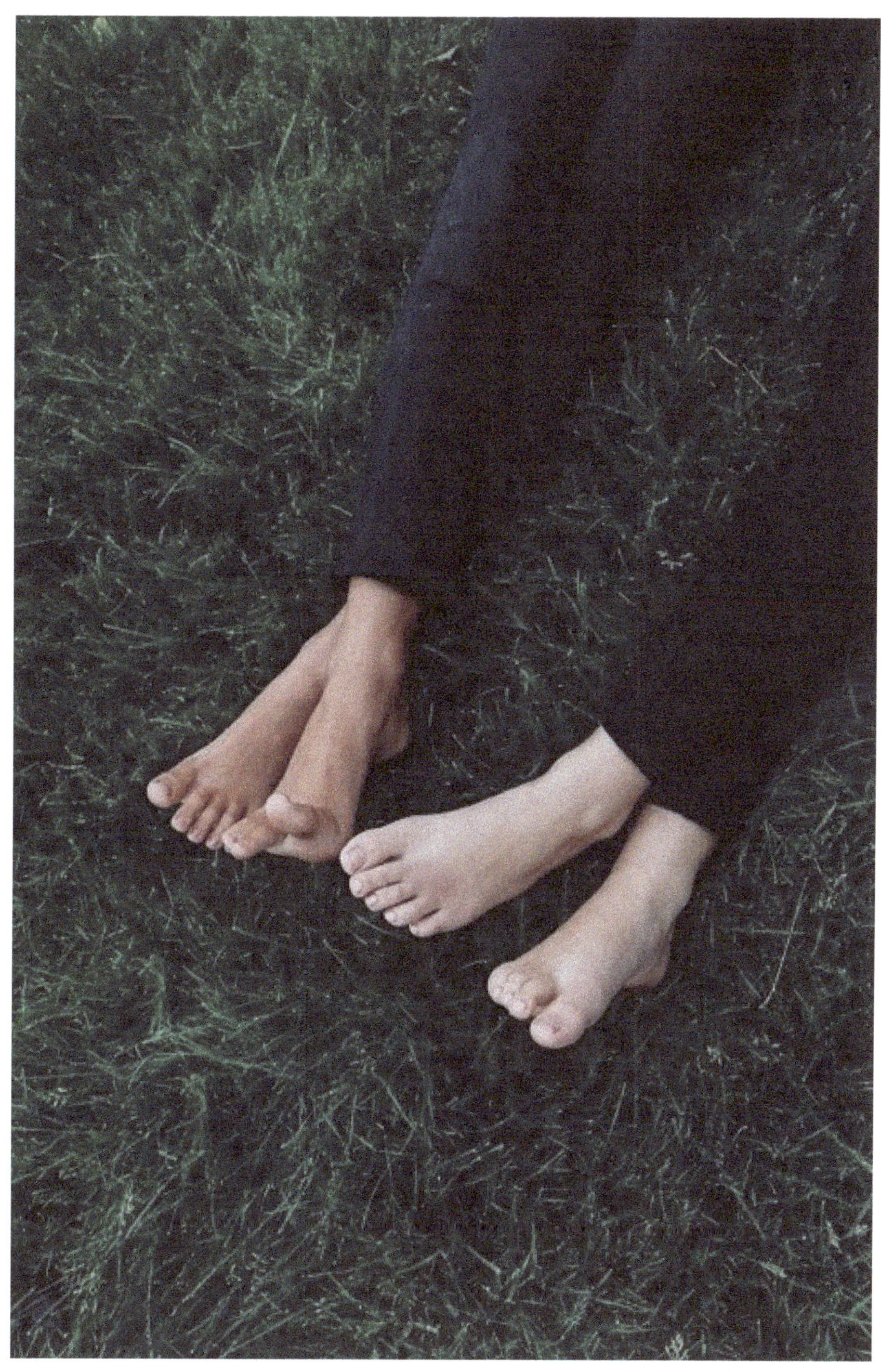

Image by Olichel from Pixabay

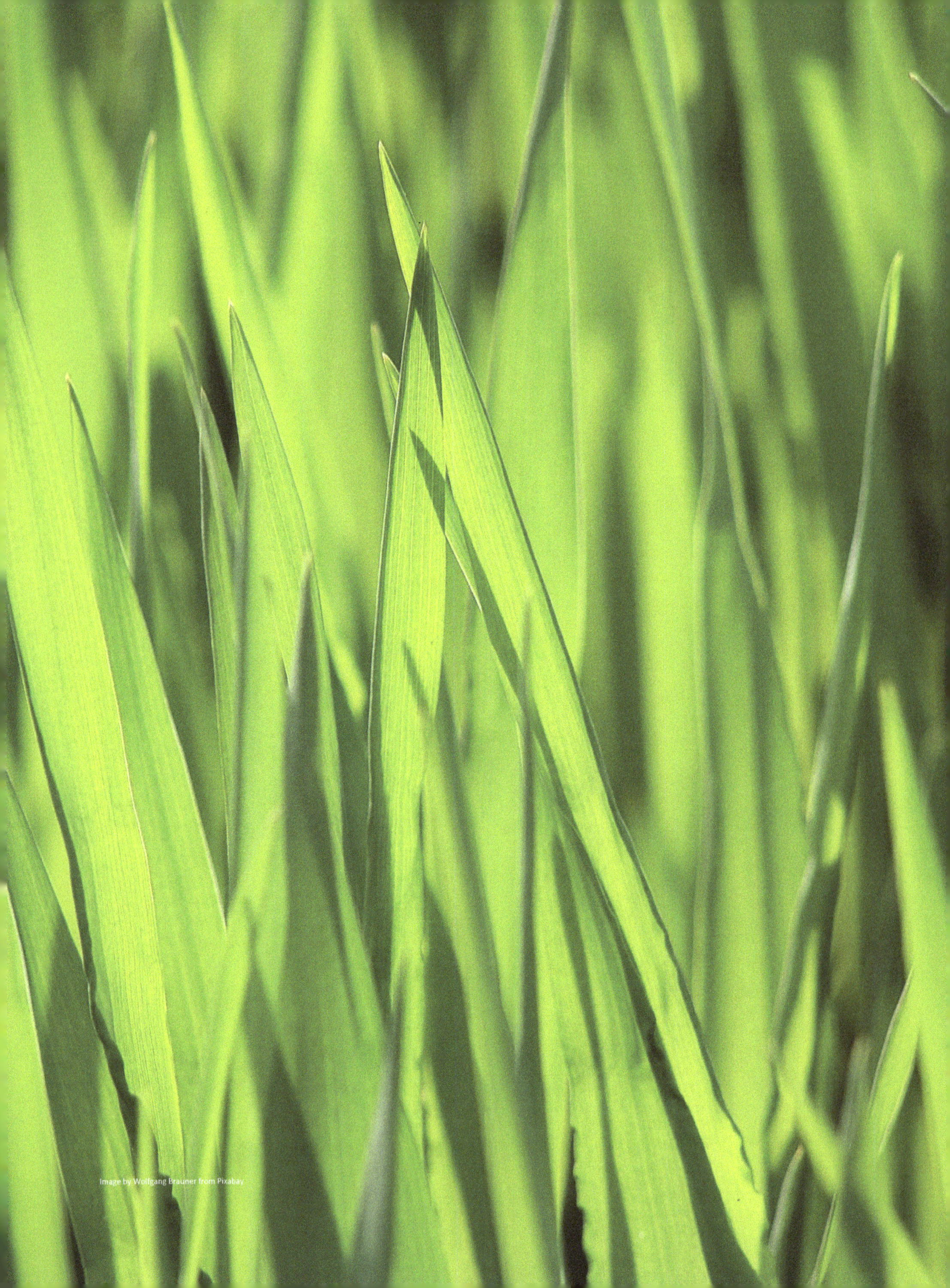

Image by Wolfgang Brauner from Pixabay

Vetiver grass - Chrysopogon zizanioides

Vetiver grass is native to India, and now grown around the world for uses such as perfumery, essential oil and as an environmental stabilising plant. The grass grows as a tight clump, and like bamboo produces other out-plantings by sending out tendril shoots. The stalks and leaves can grow up to 2 meters in height with the roots penetrating up to 2-3 meters deep. As a result, the grass is used to stabilise slopes and to revegetate, as it tolerates droughts due to the deep roots.

One of the primary uses of Vetiver grass is the oil made from the roots. This oil has been used for centuries in the perfume industry due to its woody and pungent odour. It shares many aspects with other aromatic grasses such as lemongrass. Currently, the primary producers of the oil are Haiti, India, Reunion and Indonesia. Over the last few decades, the essential oil has become a mainstay in the aromatherapy industry with many claims made as to its health benefits, but its main claim is the relaxing effect the oil has.

Early research on the oil was carried out by Dr Terry S Friedman of the United States. In his preliminary research he showed that by simply smelling the essential oil, a significant improvement was achieved in children suffering from Attention Deficit and Hyperactivity Disorder (ADHD). In his published paper he showed it a possible 32% improvement in ADHD symptoms could be achieved; an overall improvement in focus and a reduction in hyperactivity, allowing children to relax and remain attentive to classroom activities.

In its native region of India, Vetiver grass is known as Khas Khas, and has been used in Ayurvedic medicine for centuries. The plant has been used for various health applications, and its use for the central nervous system has been constant. A clinical study of the effects of the plant on anxiety and depression in 2015 found that the ethanol extract from the roots had similar actions as the standard drug fluoxetine. In this paper, the researchers also combined the extract of Vetiver with Foeniculum vulgar (fennel) and found that this combination was as effective as fluoxetine. It is believed that the anti-inflammatory actions of the plant are the main contributing factor in the reduction of depression.

Claims that Vetiver enhances memory and learning was studied in 2014, and its research found that a dose of 500 mg/kg bodyweight of the ethanolic extract from Vetiver grass did indeed increase memory and retention of information. The standard drug piracetam was used in this clinical research as a comparative control. The findings showed that the plant extract had similar actions and is therefore of interest in treating age related cognitive decline.

Additional research from 2014 sought to understand the ability of the ethanol extract from the roots in the reduction of anxiety. Once again, the outcome of the research endorsed the use of the plant in the treatment of anxiety related disorders, and it believed the responsible actions of the extract was the inhibition of acetylcholinesterase, a compound found in the body that affects the functions of neurotransmitters. The standard drug used as a control in this research was diazepam.

[1] D. Cultivation et al., "Chrysopogon zizanioides".

[2] T. S. Friedmann, "2 . 2 .," pp. 1–5.

[3] B. Bhushan, S. K. Sharma, T. Singh, L. Singh, and H. Arya, "Vetiveria Zizanioides (Linn.) Nash: a Pharmacological Overview," Int. Res. J. Pharm., vol. 4, no. 7, pp. 18–20, 2013.

[4] G. J. I, A. A. Elizabeth, K. Punnagai, N. S. Muthiah, G. Josephine, and J. C. P. Res, "Journal of Chemical and Pharmaceutical Research , 2015 , 7 (8): 729-734 Research Article Comparative study of Vetiveria zizanioides and Foeniculum vulgare extracts on behavioral despair of Wistar albino rats," vol. 7, no. 8, pp. 729–734, 2015.

[5] C. Velmurugan, S. K. Shajahan, B. S. A. Kumar, S. V. Kumar, R. A. Priyadharshini, and S. Thomas, "Memory and learning enhancing activity of different extracts of roots of Vetiveria zizanioides," Int. J. Nov. Trends Pharm. Sci., vol. 4, no. 6, pp. 174–182, 2014.

[6] A. M. Nirwane, P. V. Gupta, J. H. Shet, and S. B. Patil, "Anxiolytic and nootropic activity of Vetiveria zizanioides roots in mice," J. Ayurveda Integr. Med., vol. 6, no. 3, pp. 158–164, 2015.

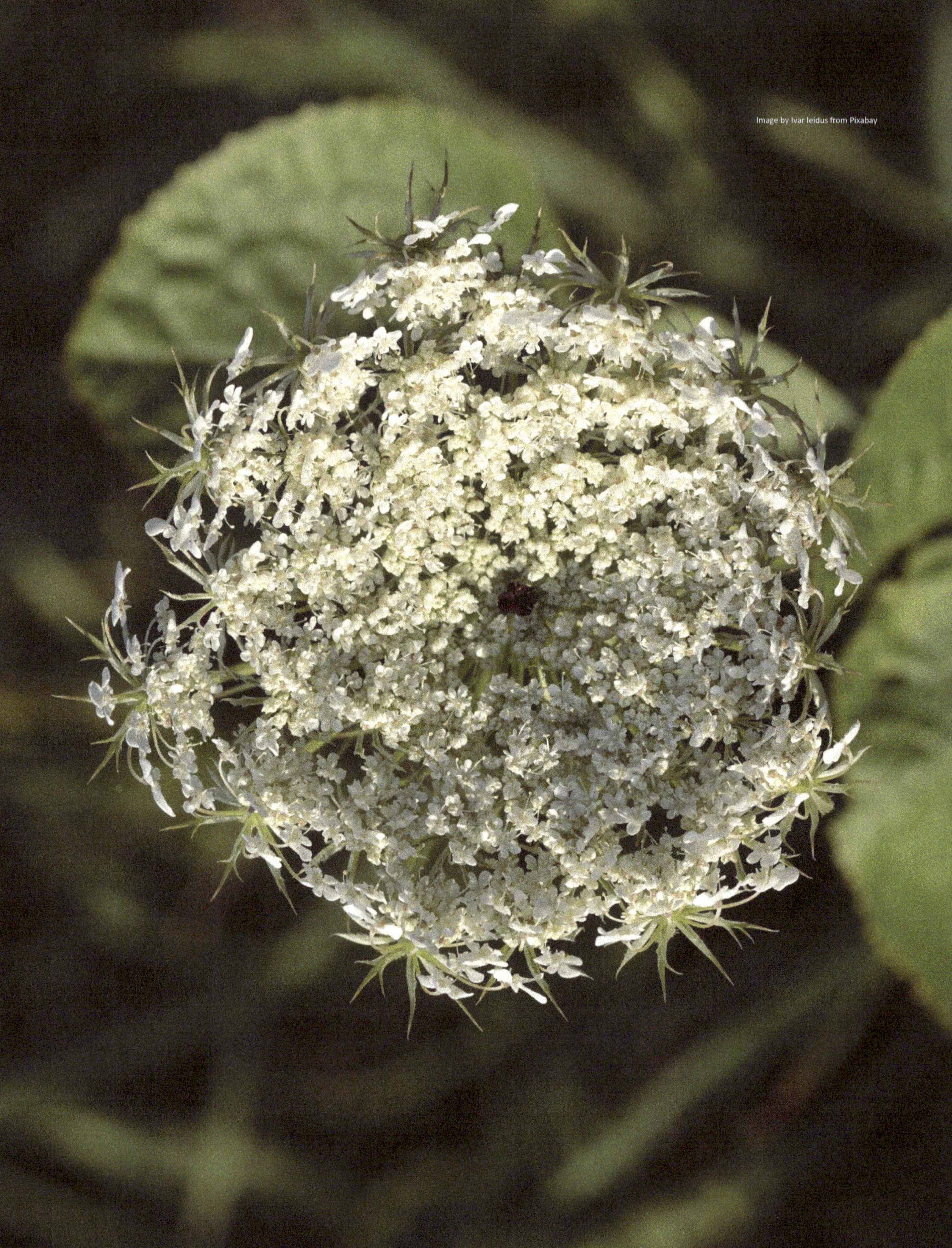

Image by Ivar leidus from Pixabay

Wild Carrot / Queens Anne Lace - Daucus carota

Wild Carrot is related to parsley, coriander, fennel, anise, dill and cumin. It is the forebear of the modern-day carrot and is thought to have originated in Afghanistan. The plant has a long history. It is believed to have been in use for the past 2 or 3,000 years primarily for the flowers, seeds and leaves rather than the tuber as it is nowadays. Its medicinal qualities were first used, and they have been recorded as such in both Greek and Roman texts.

It is an unassuming plant that is a member of the Apiaceae family. It can easily be confused with Poison Hemlock, so care must be taken when trying to collect it from the wild. As a medicinal herb, it is a surprising inclusion here as it is primarily thought of as a vegetable. The seeds however are the most important part of the plant in the preparation of either the essential oil or ethanolic extract.

A review of the Wild Carrot's therapeutic application from 2017 lists the following uses of the herb ranging from antioxidant, hypotensive, hepatoprotective, nephroprotective, antidiabetic, memory enhancing, antimicrobial, antidepressant, and others. We are focused here on the neuroprotective, anxiolytic and antidepressant claims which fortunately have been widely studied. Significant findings were revealed in research into the neuroprotective and improvements in cognitive functions, via the use of the ethanol extract derived from the seeds of Daucus carota. Improvements in memory were recorded in both young and aged mice in the laboratory. Increments of 23% improvement at doses of 200 mg/kg body weight, and 35% at doses of 400 mg/kg body weight over a ten-day period. There was a significant reduction in brain cholesterol and acetylcholinesterase. In young mice the cholesterol levels were reduced by 23%, and 21% in aged mice. The acetylcholinesterase levels were reduced by 22% in young mice, and 19% in aged mice. Acetylcholinesterase is an enzyme that breaks down various neurotransmitters in the body, and a reduction in this enzyme will positively elevate nerve function. The findings from the reviewed research stated that the results show that Daucus carota may be an important adjunct to the treatment of Alzheimer's disease and other forms of dementia.

Citing research from 2014, the review also quoted research from 2000 that showed the ethanolic extract from the roots of the plant at doses of 400 mg/kg body weight displayed significant antidepressant effects that were comparable to the standard drugs fluoxetine and desipramine. The seeds are reported to contain high levels of choline which may be one of the active compounds in studied effects.

Research from 2009 showed that the plant is also a potent anti-inflammatory and that it displays anti-inflammatory effects up to 50%+ in inflammation modelling. This piece of research used the ethanol extract derived from the flowers or umbels. Other research into the anti-inflammatory potential of Wild Carrot used the ethanol extract of the seeds, and also showed a measurable reduction in the histamine response. It even showed a reduction in prostaglandins associated with inflammatory reactions within the body. Therefore, the potential for Daucus carota to reduce inflammatory conditions in the brain is supported in clinical research as well as the resulting reduction in anxiety and depression.

[1] P. D. A. E. Al-Snafi, "Nutritional and therapeutic importance of Daucus carota- A review," IOSR J. Pharm., vol. 07, no. 02, pp. 72–88, 2017.

[2] Q. Anne et al., "Daucus carota."

[3] P. N. Babu, B. Nagaraju, K. Yamini, M. Dhananjaneyulu, K. Venkateswarlu, and M. Mubina, "Evaluation of antidepressant activity of ethanolic extract of Dacus carota in mice," J. Pharm. Sci. Res., vol. 6, no. 2, pp. 73–77, 2014.

[4] R. Bahrami, A. Ghobadi, N. Behnoud, and E. Akhtari, "Medicinal Properties of Daucus carota in Traditional Persian Medicine and Modern Phytotherapy," pp. 107–114, 2018.

Religion the great antidepressant

"Do not pray for an easy life. Pray for the strength to endure a difficult one"

Bruce Lee

One of the hallmarks of depression is emptiness, of being lost in your own head and at the whim of futility. Dark thoughts and unanswered questions abound; "Why am I not good enough?", "What is the point?", and "What does it all mean?" are just some examples. For some people, it is all too much and having someone or something give you all the answers is more than tempting. The surrender to a higher power and nicely packaged purpose is comfortable. No more questions, just a simple faith can be rewarding.

At the beginning of the evolution of religions, it was the external world that devotees wanted answers for. All manner of things were blamed on a plethora of Gods. A storm at sea; blame it on Neptune or Poseidon. For a famine, we can blame it on Ganesh or Ceres. A disease; blame it on Wen-Shen or Apollo. War, well you can pray to Mars or Freyja or Gurzil for a positive outcome. There was a god for any occasion, and we submitted to their whimsical natures even though we can ascertain they did not physically or actually exist. We could abdicate our own responsibilities and blame, foisting them onto any suitable god. This worked well for a while and gods were invented and then replaced by better ones over time until certain prophets and messiahs streamlined the entire process to a one stop one god shop. So today there are only a few god's, but they control everything. The Hindu religion is one of the few still surviving today with a multitude of gods, however they all originate from one all-powerful deity.

Today there are twelve main religions. These are in order of oldest to youngest as Hinduism, Judaism, Jainism, Shinto, Zoroastrianism, Buddhism, Taoism, Confucianism, Christianity, Islam, Sikhism and Baha'i. The Encyclopaedia Britannica states "Religion, is defined as human being's relation to that which they regard as holy, sacred, absolute, spiritual, divine, or worthy of especial reverence." So, a structured belief system regulating behaviour and thought, and if followed rigorously, removed any questions and doubt about life and death. In short, an acceptance of a meaning for life, where before there was none. There was only depression.

A recent paper from Canada reviewed a multitude of research papers into the correlation between the decrease of depression and religious communities, groups, or individuals. It comes as no surprise that there was a substantial decrease in depression, anxiety and negative psychological conditions when people submitted to a religious ideal. All 105 research papers identified as possible inclusion in the meta-analysis, yet only 23 were eligible or more precisely, robust enough to draw usable data from. Needless to say, we must assume that the authors of the research papers are not themselves religious fanatics and their findings are unbiased. As a result, whilst we find that religion is a panacea for the lost soul, the question here is how it came about. No pharmaceutical can claim such impressive results as kneeling in a basement on cold winter mornings can. So, we must accept the premise that religious people are far less depressed than non-religious people. However, this is not so simple. First, we have to look at how these religions came into being. Who was behind them and what sort of mental state were they in at the time? We have to psychoanalyze the chicken in order to understand the egg.

Of the world's twelve main religions Buddhism is the fourth largest with approximately 520 million adherents. The founder of this school of spiritual thought never wanted his works to end up as a religion, yet it has become so for varying reasons such as traditions, ceremony, and group identity. These will become clearer later. First, we need to look at Siddhartha Gautama, the young prince who became the Buddha. It is no small leap to assume that when you are happy you wish to remain so for as long as you can. Yet misery and unhappiness push you to change. This can be applied to Siddhartha when he sneaked out of his father's palace one evening, leaving behind his wife and son so that he could live the life of a monk or aesthetic with only a loincloth and a begging bowl. Siddhartha wanted above all to understand life and to find a way to avoid pain and suffering. This should sound familiar to the majority of people suffering from depression.

Siddhartha practised meditation and extreme denial of all pleasures for several years until he realised that he still had not found release from the misery of life. It was this realisation that made him decide to sit under the Peepal tree (Ficus religiosa) and not move until he had achieved enlightenment. During his time under the tree in deep meditation, the story relates how he was tempted by Mara the Lord of the Desire realm who sent his daughters to seduce the young monk. This temptation theme is common to both Christianity as well as Islam. As with Christ and Mohammed, Siddhartha refused to be tempted and thereby attained enlightenment. He became free from depression and pain. Therefore, before he sat under the Bodhi tree Buddha was wracked with uncertainty and unhappiness and directly afterwards no longer suffered from either of them. What happened next has created an enormous amount of debate over the centuries. Shortly after arising as the new Buddha, Siddhartha, refused to teach anyone his method of enlightenment as he thought that people would not understand him as they were too caught up in worldliness.

The Holy Prophet Mohammad was also wracked by depression and thoughts of suicide. It is well known that the Holy prophet spent long periods of time in a cave isolated from others while he considered his life and its meaning. Jesus also spent his famous forty days fasting in the desert and fighting with Satan. In all the Prophet Mohammad spent thirty days in his cave, Jesus forty days in the desert, and Buddha spent forty-nine days under a tree. Other religions and their founders follow similar patterns of emotional turmoil as is the case with Joseph Smith the founder of Mormonism. So, religion it appears can be seen as a product or answer to the questioning depressed soul, and it is relatively easy today to find sermons and lectures from these religious systems on how to deal with depression by simply accepting the teaching professed in them. It is interesting to note in this discussion that all religions consider suicide to be a sin, which is particularly relevant in regard to a system or systems that arose from how best to deal with depression.

Becoming a devotee of religion however may not be suitable for everyone, for various reasons. Nonetheless, we can gain insights from religious practice such as acceptance. The simple act of joining a religion requires acceptance or faith in their teachings and answers that the religion of choice has created for its followers. One aspect of depression is the almost eternal internal questioning a sufferer has about themselves, the world, and their place in it. How tempting it would be to replace these questions of self-worth with blind faith, and, if possible, simply accept that you are depressed and get on with life no matter how grey it may be. Similar to Alcoholics Anonymous meetings that require as the first step the admission that you are indeed an alcoholic. Without this first step in accepting your problem, no further improvement is possible.

Another aspect of religious practice is belonging to a likeminded community or group. If there was actually one health crisis that should have no problem with creating a community or group, then that is depression. With so many people around the world suffering from the condition, it is a unique trait of feeling depressed to have the feeling of being so alone and isolated, and yet having so many members with the same affliction in common. The lesson here is to refrain from isolating yourself, by either joining a discussion group on depression or less threatening, any club or association.

The implied or even overt message from religion is a 'sense of purpose or reason for existence'. All religions impel their adherents to work to attain membership in a goal or ideal such as heaven, Valhalla or Nirvana. Whilst these may be too esoteric for the common run of the mill depressed person, a simple decision to excel at a skill or art may be just as good.

In a nutshell, if there was a religion called the Depressed Church of the Holy Black Poodle it would have the following commandments:

One	Accept your depression.
Two	Get together with other disciples of depression.
Three	Your purpose of life is to channel depression into art, sport, a hobby, and helping others with depression.

A religion with only three commandments.

If you wish to know what perfect devotion and faith look like, then look at your dog.

[1] A. A. Mahdanian, "Journal of Psychiatry and Behavioral Health Forecast Religion and Depression : A Review of the Literature," vol. 1, no. March, pp. 1–4, 2018.

[2] R. Bonelli, R. E. Dew, H. G. Koenig, D. H. Rosmarin, and S. Vasegh, "Religious and spiritual factors in depression: Review and integration of the research," *Depress. Res. Treat.*, vol. 2012, 2012.

[3] M. Zuckerman, J. Silberman, and J. A. Hall, "The Relation Between Intelligence and Religiosity: A Meta-Analysis and Some Proposed Explanations," *Personal. Soc. Psychol. Rev.*, vol. 17, no. 4, pp. 325–354, 2013.

[4] J. Sickles, A. Huskey, K. Schrantz, and C. W. Lack, "The Relationship between Intelligence and Religiosity : A Critical Review of the Literature," *J. Sci. Psychol.*, no. May, pp. 1–10, 2015.

[5] E. D. Murray, M. G. Cunningham, and B. H. Price, "The role of psychotic disorders in religious history considered," *J. Neuropsychiatry Clin. Neurosci.*, vol. 24, no. 4, pp. 410–426, 2012.

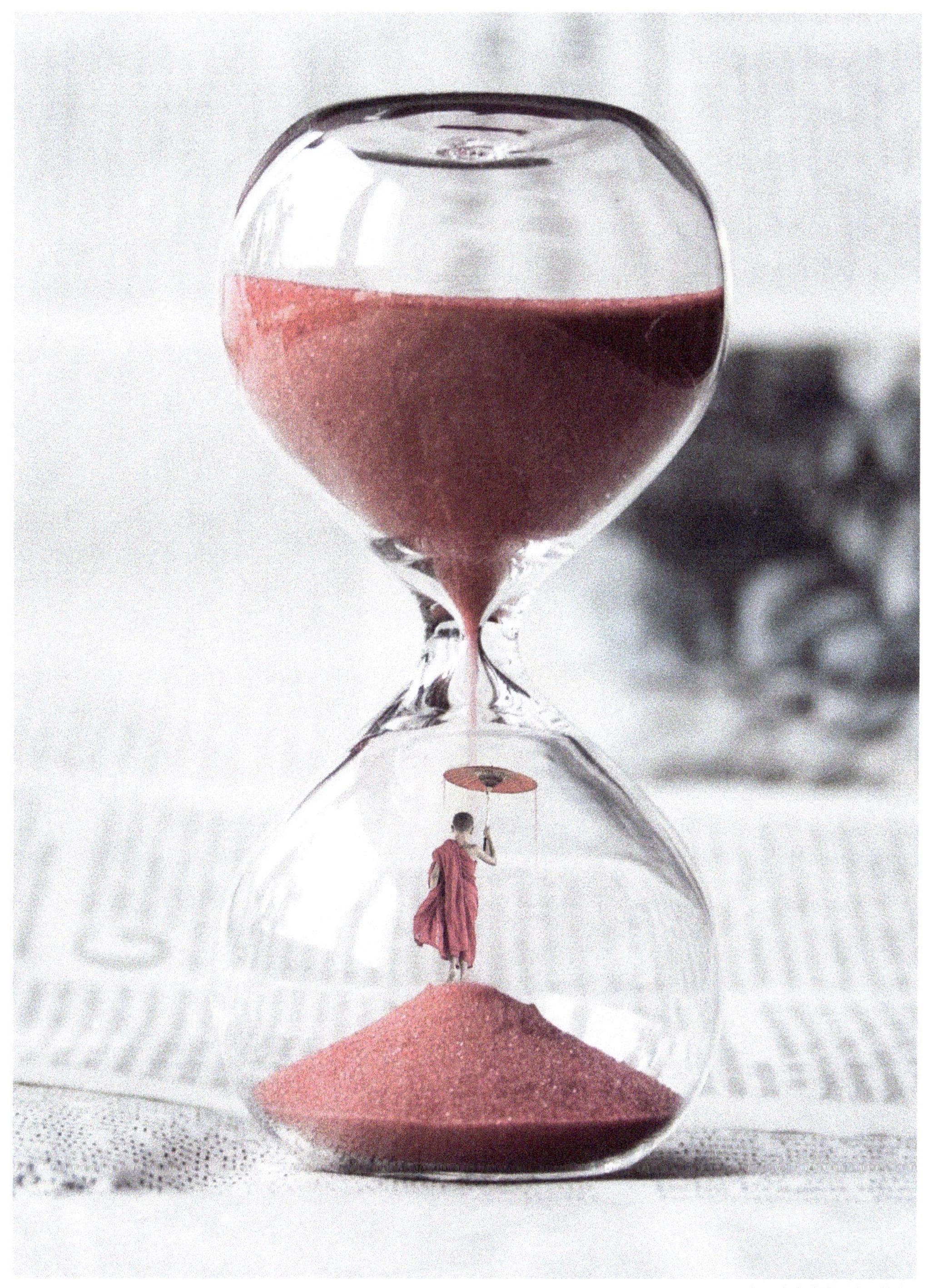

Image by Funky Focus from Pixabay

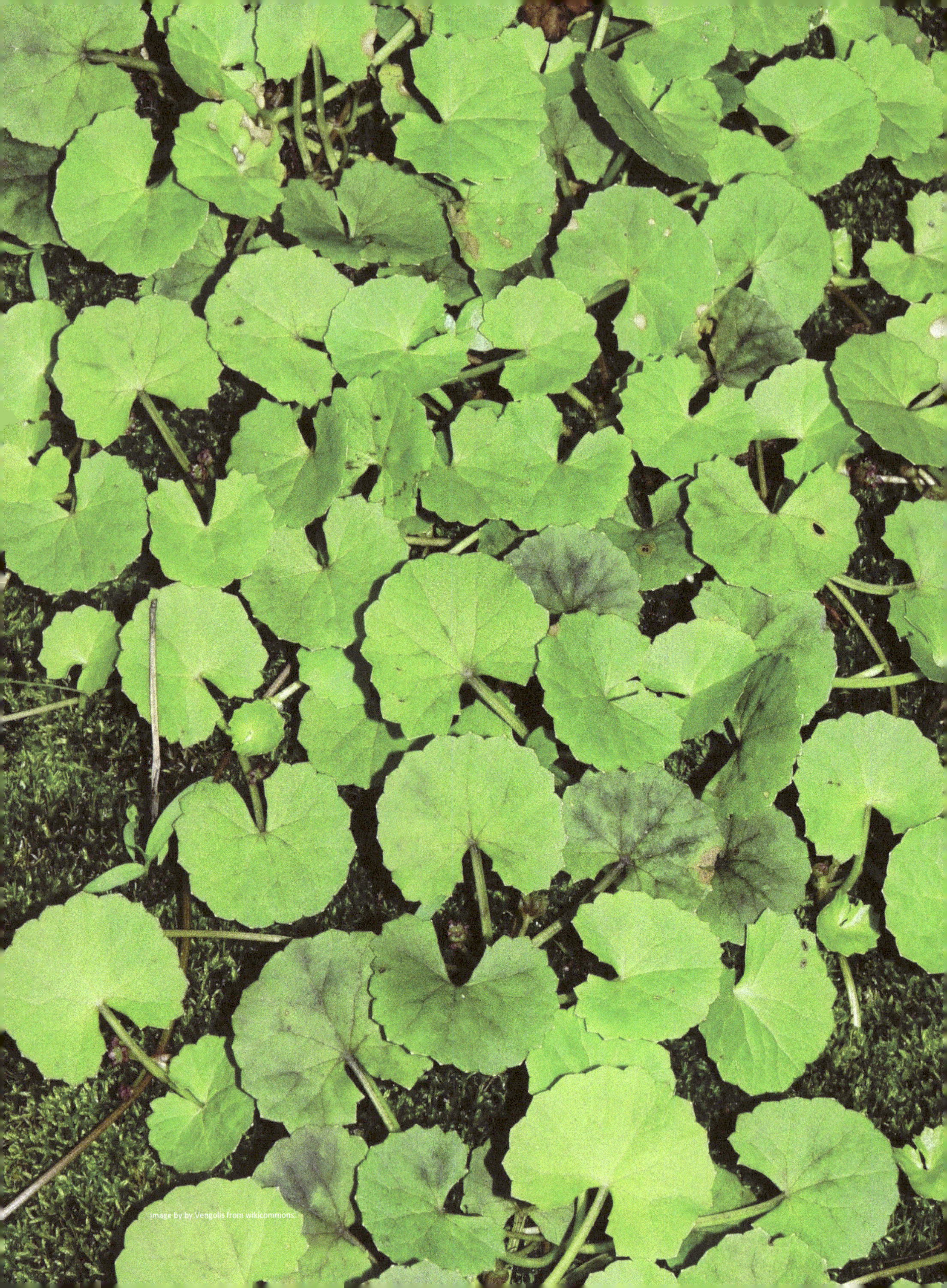

Image by by Vengolis from wikicommons.

Pennywort - Centella asiatica

Centella asiatica is a low growing plant found in tropical zones around the world. Primarily used in Asia in both cuisines as a salad item and the traditional medicine systems of the region. The herb has grown in popularity of the last few decades as a general tonic. It is claimed to aid in the treatment of specific health disorders, and acts as a cardiotonic, nerve tonic, sedative to nerves, stomachic, carminative, improves appetite, antileprotic, memory and reduces fever. As stated with Bacopa monnieri, there is a double use of the common name, Brahmi herb, for both.

A great deal of research has been conducted on the plant, and its antidepressant actions have been endorsed, but not well understood.

In one clinical trial, the extract from Pennywort was combined with the standard antidepressant drug known as venlafaxine. This study from 2013 sought to understand the possible combination therapies that may be more beneficial for sufferers of depression. Venlafaxine is a novel antidepressant as it works on both the norepinephrine and serotonin monoamines and far less on the dopamine levels. The results from this study showed that Centella asiatica amplified the benefits achieved from the use of venlafaxine, yet Centella by itself did not have significant results at 100 mg/kg body weight. While this report shows the benefit of combination therapies, the dose used for Centella asiatica may have been too small to have any real effect on the test subjects.

Another study from 2012 used low doses of Centella asiatica over a period of 14 days and did show improvements in the symptoms of depression. Therefore, the use of the herb may take 10 to 14 days of use before any improvement is felt by the sufferer, which may explain the poor result of only Centella asiatica in the 2013 study.

The triterpenoid glycosides, including madecassic acid, asiatic acid, madecassoside, and asiaticoside, are the most active compounds isolated from Centella asiatica. In a study into the protective effects derived from the plant, fluoxetine was used as the standard drug comparative. In this study, it was shown that doses of up to 800 mg/kg body weight had similar results to that of fluoxetine. As can be seen, the 2013 study used doses of 100 mg/kg body weight, which is far lower than the one being discussed here. The results from this study were collated after 8 weeks, and a significant reduction in stress, anxiety and depression was observed. In addition to these benefits, it has also been shown that the use of the herb over time protects against neuronal damage and therefore protects memory and cognitive function in test subjects.

Adding Pennywort to your salads may be a nice change, however it will not deliver the necessary dose to have any long-term benefit. Nonetheless, you will have a unique salad.

[1] V. Kumar, A. Tomar, B. K. Singh, K. Nagarajan, L. Machawal, and U. Bajaj, "Attenuating depression behaviour by Centella asiatica extract & venlafaxine in mice induced through Forced swim and Tail suspension test," Int. J. Pharmacol. Toxicol., vol. 1, no. 2, 2013.

[2] Z. Navratilova and J. Patocka, "[Centela asiatica, a medicinal plant with anxiolytic, antidepressant and neuroprotective effects]," no. November 2015, 2014.

[3] G. Kola et al., "Centella asiatica," pp. 5–8.

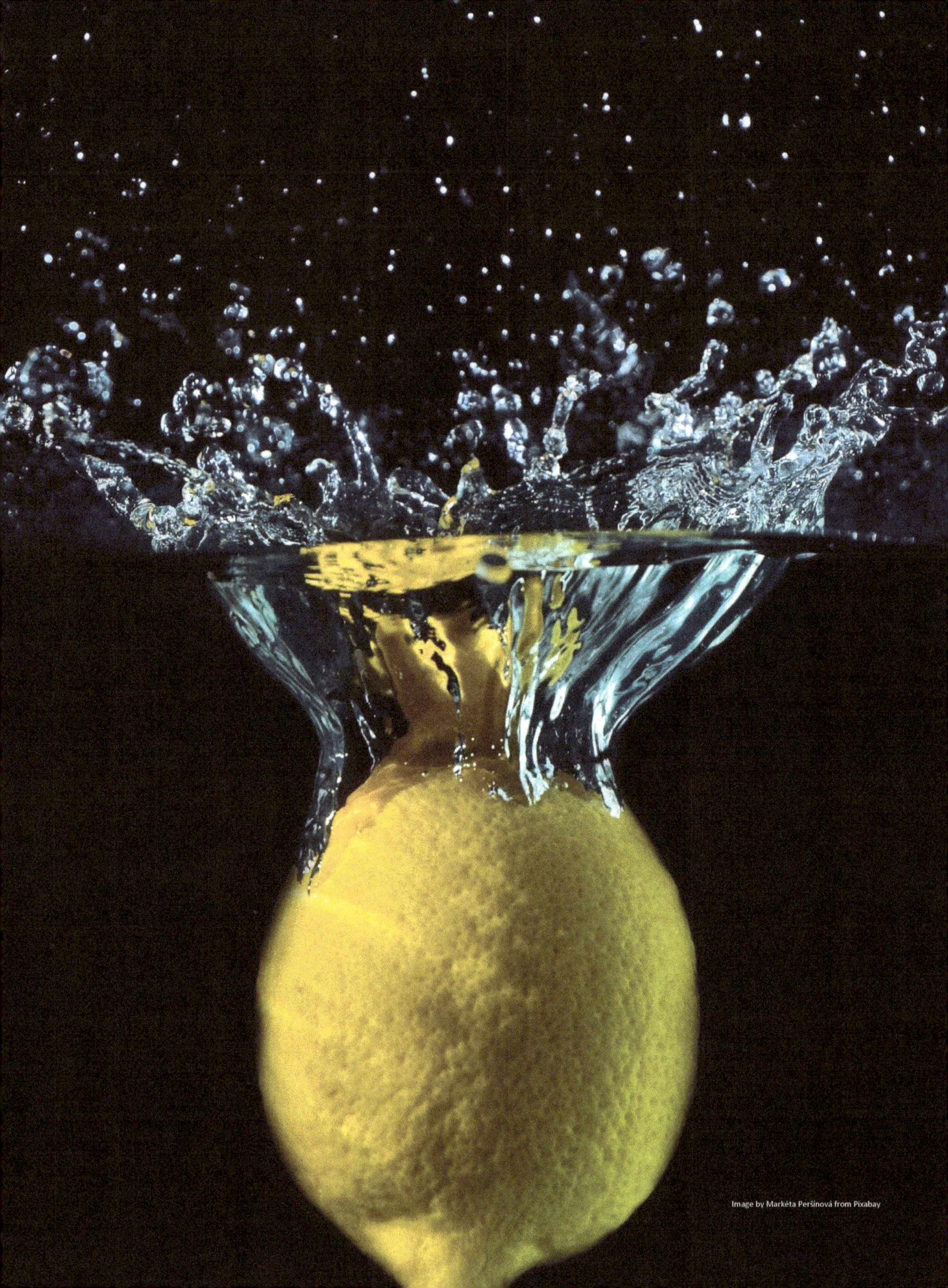

Image by Markéta Peršinová from Pixabay

Lemon - Citrus limon

The staple addition to a Gin and Tonic, the lemon is one of the most widely grown fruits in the world. It is believed that they originated from central Asia near Burma, Northern India and China. From here they were introduced into ancient Rome in the second century A.D. Today lemons are used in perfumery, to flavour food and drinks, and also as medicine.

The juice from lemon has high levels of citric acid and has a pH of around 2.2. It also contains high levels of ascorbic acid (vitamin C) , as a 100-gram serving of lemon may deliver up to 64% of a person's daily need. Lemon juice as a medicine is used to actually raise the pH of the body into a more alkaline state. This is indeed contraindicative, as the lemon in its natural state is acidic, but when it is ingested, it aids in making the gut more alkaline.

The most common product used in alternative health circles is the oil of the lemon tree. This oil is either derived from the leaves or from the skin of the fruit. A common use for the oil is as an aromatherapy agent where it has been shown to increase concentration, productivity, and mood. It is the research into the anti-anxiety and anti-depressive actions of the oil that are surprising.

In a study conducted in China in 2012, researchers showed that oral doses of lemon oil up to 800 mg/kg body weight created significant improvement in mice without side effects. In this trial, the lemon oil was compared to the standard anti-depression drug fluoxetine. The outcome showed that whilst lemon oil was significant, it was not as effective as fluoxetine. However, there was an increase in dopamine and serotonin activity, indicating a very real and useful adjunct in the treatment of depression.

A Brazilian study into the calming effects of a lemon extract made from the leaves was also positive. In this trial, conducted in 2013, the ethanol extract from the leaves was compared to diazepam, imipramine and paroxetine. They are all standard antidepressant medications. It was found that at doses of 150 mg/kg body weight, the lemon extract outperformed all three synthetic drugs, and when combined with them amplified their effects.

Finally, and in support of the aromatherapy claims made on the essential oil made from the peel of the lemon fruit, a trial (2015) also from Brazil, showed that the simple inhalation of the aroma had significant improvement in depression models. It was found that when the inhalation of the aroma of the oil occurred, a considerable improvement in anxiety models was witnessed, however it was not as effective as the standard drug known as diazepam. The aroma from the oil of the lemon peel had a positive effect on sleep patterns as well.

So, if you meet someone strongly smelling of lemons, be kind as they might just be suffering from depression.

[1] C. W. Hao, W. S. Lai, C. T. Ho, and L. Y. Sheen, "Antidepressant-like effect of lemon essential oil is through a modulation in the levels of norepinephrine, dopamine, and serotonin in mice: Use of the tail suspension test," J. Funct. Foods, vol. 5, no. 1, pp. 370–379, 2013.

[2] et al., "Anxiolytic- and antidepressant-like effects of the ethanolic extract from Citrus limon plant widely used in Northeastern Brazil," African J. Pharm. Pharmacol., vol. 7, no. 30, pp. 2173–2179, 2013.

[3] M. D. M. VIANA et al., "Anxiolytic-like effect of Citrus limon (L.) Burm f. essential oil inhalation on mice," Rev. Bras. Plantas Med., vol. 18, no. 1, pp. 96–104, 2016.

[4] S. Asia et al., "The lemon".

The test you need to fail!

"Man makes plans ....and God laughs"

Michael Chabon

There is a saying that "If it cannot be measured, it cannot be managed." Often used in business management, this statement is also true of the sciences. However, how can you measure emptiness when it is not contained by any walls. How is it possible to weigh a soul?

It will come as no surprise to know that therapists and doctors worldwide try to do this every day. In clinics, medical centers, hospitals, and psychiatric wards, a variety of tests are employed with the express aim of measuring a person's happiness. Science has cut out and placed on scales the human heart to find that the mean weight of the heart is 280-340 g in males and 230-280 g in females. Yet how many grams is the average happiness? This all sounds so ridiculous and implausible, and in many ways it is. However, when we look at the clinical tests for depression, the term 'ridiculous' takes on a life of its own.

One of the first rating scales for depression was developed by Dr Max Hamilton in 1960 and is still being used today for some strange reason. The next is the Beck Depression Rating Inventory developed by Aaron Beck in 1961, who went on to develop the Beck Anxiety Inventory, Beck Hopelessness Scale, Beck Suicidal Ideation Rating, and the Clark-Beck Obsessive-Compulsive Inventory. Most are under copyright and therefore make money out of rating another person's pain and suffering. This would not be so sad if they were more in tune with actual depression, or the reality they are trying to measure. Strangely both Max's and Aaron's questionnaires use 21 questions. What this means we are not really sure, however the questionnaires share some striking similarities. They start with the basics, with the first question rating how sad you are. Such a condescending start bodes unwell for the rest of the questions. Max in his Hamilton Scale takes an interest in burping and farting, whereas Aaron in his Beck Inventory is fascinated by crying. Both have a keen interest in a person's libido or lack of it, which raises concerns as science still had not discovered the full power of the clitoris by 1961. It is disconcerting that at the time that Max and Aaron developed their questionnaires, the barbarity of cutting the brain of a living person in half, known as lobotomy, was quite popular as a treatment for psychiatric disorders. Even more disconcerting was the majority of victims subjected to this cruel medical procedure were women. A 1951 study of American hospitals found nearly 60% of lobotomy patients were women; limited data shows 74% of lobotomies in Ontario from 1948–1952 were performed on women. The main differentiating aspects between Max and Aaron is that the Hamilton Depression Scale is designed for the clinician or doctor to complete, whilst Aaron decided his would be filled in by the patient. The obvious danger in both is the interpretation by the therapist and or clinician who, pending on the circumstances, may be able to commit a person to long term therapy against their will or, as we have seen, a surgical procedure.

On further shallow analysis, why would a person think that fame and fortune would be theirs if they nailed their name to an inane list of questions merely asking if a person is happy or not? Happily for Max and Aaron, they were not alone as Weinberg, Zung, Rosenberg, and others all strangely did the same. Yet, where during all of this period were the mothers? The carers? The nurturers? Why was this time of therapy dominated by men? More disturbing, is why after considering these simple influences such as time, gender, and current science, are we still using these scales today?

Many other individuals and institutions have developed their own rating scales in the attempt to define or achieve a diagnosis of depression. Some are comprehensive and ask a plethora of questions. Some are puerile, asking a seemingly bare minimum number as is the case with the Patient Health Questionnaire, better known as the 'PHQ-9'. It asks nine questions, six of which are irrelevant after the initial two that ascertain if you feel depressed and take no pleasure in life. Once you have answered the most basic and patently obvious questions "Are you depressed?" and if so, "How long have you felt this way?" If the answer to the second question is longer than a few weeks, then it is highly probable that you are indeed depressed. All that is then required is to ascertain how critical the situation is by asking "Have you thought of suicide?" If the answer is negative, then we have time to explore the how's and why's. However, if the answer is a "Yes", then a more proactive approach will be required. This simplistic diagnosis allows for the appreciation that no two people share precisely the same view of their depressions. For example, if we go back to Max and Aaron and their interest in low libido, we find that they had a complete disregard for someone who displays an overactive libido which may be an attempt for acceptance and desirability. We need to allow or accept each person to be an individual, and in so doing, depression, as an emotional state, will be unique to each person.

There do exist some scales that are far superior to the others exist that are much easier to recommend here. One such scale is the Minnesota Multiphasic Personality Inventory (MMP-2) which is comprised of in excess of three hundred questions that are reviewed and updated on a much better timeframe than many others. Though who's idea was it to use the term 'inventory' anyway, and why?

In certain circumstances the rating scales and inventories may also prove useful. Such as in a situation where a person is in denial about their emotional state and may find a better understanding or clarity by completing an impartial set of questions.

It may seem a bit too simple and logical to ask the person if they are actually depressed. After all, if you are using a clinical set of questions, then you are most probably a therapist of some sort and not catching up with friends at a bar. It may be a wild assumption that the person answering your questions has made an appointment with you about their feelings of emptiness and sadness. It may just be a wild hunch, but if they came to your office or clinic, then they were not feeling very peachy to begin with, and after asking them a set of puerile and patently condescending questions, they may appear even more depressed than when they walked through your doors. Where are the questions on environment, the questions on family, the questions on intimacy, on whether there has been loss or trauma? Where, finally, are the insights into what depression really is?

Perhaps this is one aspect of why people do not share their feelings about being depressed. Perhaps here we see the disconnect where people are labelled as sick or unwell by medical practitioners, thereby creating negative stigmas with friends and family. In effect isolating the person even more. Depression is not contained in a set of questions. It is an experience that changes and adapts. Depression is not static. It evolves. The misogynistic, condescending and inane questions developed over half a century ago have absolutely no place in modern therapy and can be argued had no place as therapeutic tools even in 1961.

The current use of rating scales or inventories is summed up in the Abraham Maslow quote; "If you only have a hammer, you tend to see every problem as a nail!" Depression is a multifaceted condition that is influenced by diet, environment, social interactions, intelligence and more. Nevertheless, at the heart of every depressed person is a soul. A spirit that is much larger and vastly more complex than twenty-one questions.

Some of the more prominent questionnaires are as follows.

1. Beck Depression Inventory (BDI)
2. Beck Hopelessness Scale
3. Centre for Epidemiological Studies - Depression Scale (CES-D)
4. Center for Epidemiological Studies Depression Scale for Children (CES-DC)
5. Edinburgh Postnatal Depression Scale (EPDS)
6. Geriatric Depression Scale (GDS)
7. Hamilton Rating Scale for Depression (HAM-D)
8. Hospital Anxiety and Depression Scale
9. Kutcher Adolescent Depression Scale (KADS)
10. Major Depression Inventory (MDI)
11. Montgomery-Åsberg Depression Rating Scale (MADRS)
12. PHQ-9
13. Mood and Feelings Questionnaire (MFQ)
14. Weinberg Screen Affective Scale (WSAS)
15. Zung Self-Rating Depression Scale
16. Depression Anxiety Stress Scale (DASS)

Besides the best therapist and judge of character has fur and four feet.

[1] Q. Liu, H. He, J. Yang, X. Feng, F. Zhao, and J. Lyu, "Changes in the global burden of depression from 1990 to 2017: Findings from the Global Burden of Disease study," J. Psychiatr. Res., vol. 126, no. August 2019, pp. 134–140, 2019.

[2] Tagalidou, E. Distlberger, V. Loderer, and A. R. Laireiter, "Efficacy and feasibility of a humor training for people suffering from depression, anxiety, and adjustment disorder: A randomized controlled trial," BMC Psychiatry, vol. 19, no. 1, pp. 1–13, 2019.

[3] U. Willinger et al., "Cognitive and emotional demands of black humour processing: the role of intelligence, aggressiveness and mood," Cogn. Process., vol. 18, no. 2, pp. 159–167, 2017.

[4] 北村純一 et al., "1. 顔面麻痺タイプの診断に難渋した1症例 (第1回 日本リハビリテーション医学会関東地方会)," Japanese J. Rehabil. Med., vol. 34, no. 3, pp. 234–235, 1997.

[5] Johnson, Jenell (17 October 2014). American Lobotomy: A Rhetorical History. University of Michigan Press. pp. 50–60. ISBN 978-0472119448. Retrieved 12 August 2017.

[6] El-Hai, Jack (21 December 2016). "Race and Gender in the Selection of Patients for Lobotomy". Wonders & Marvels. Retrieved 12 August 2017.

[7] "Lobotomies". Western University. Retrieved 12 August 2017.

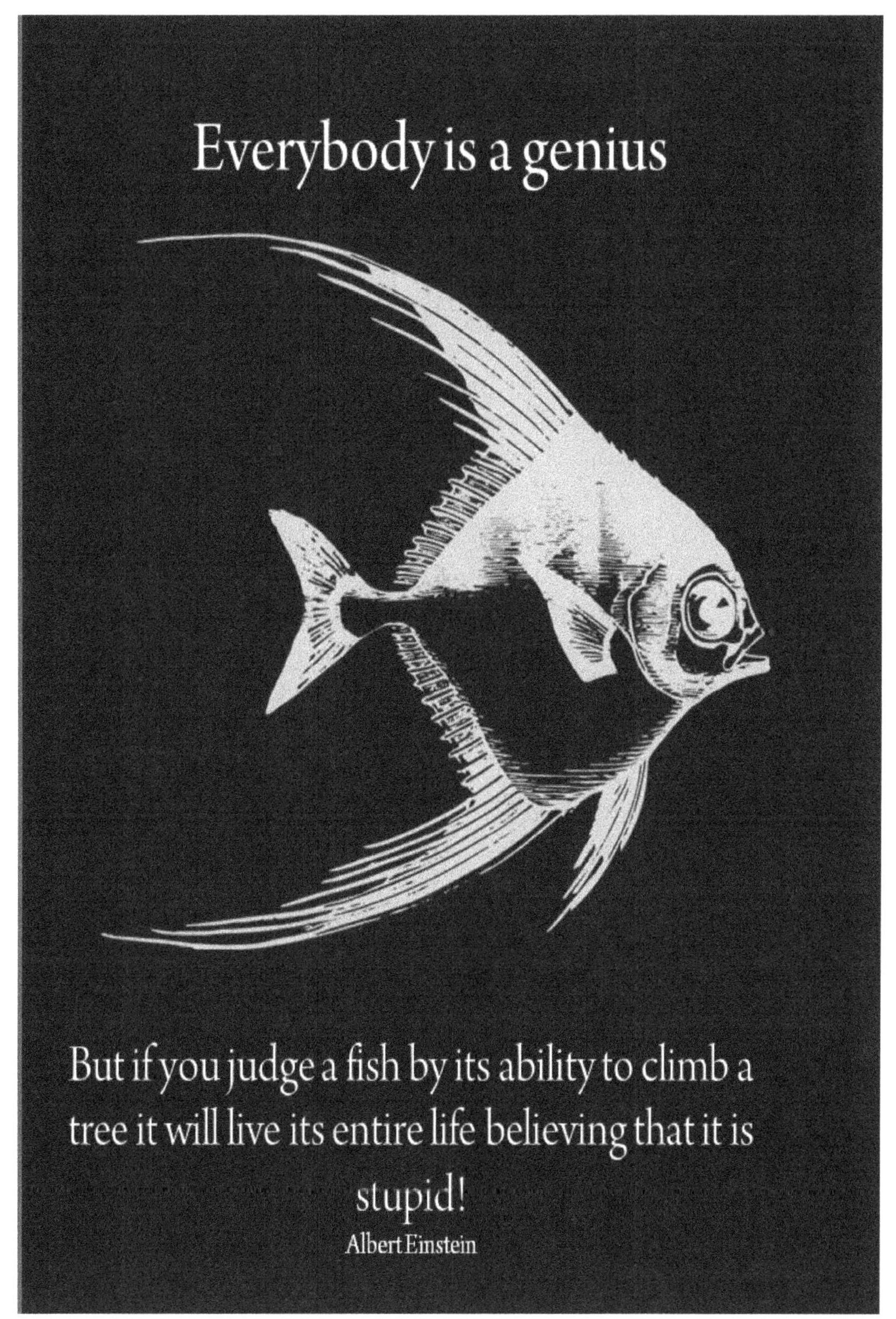
Everybody is a genius
But if you judge a fish by its ability to climb a tree it will live its entire life believing that it is stupid!
Albert Einstein

Image by Colleen ODell from Pixabay

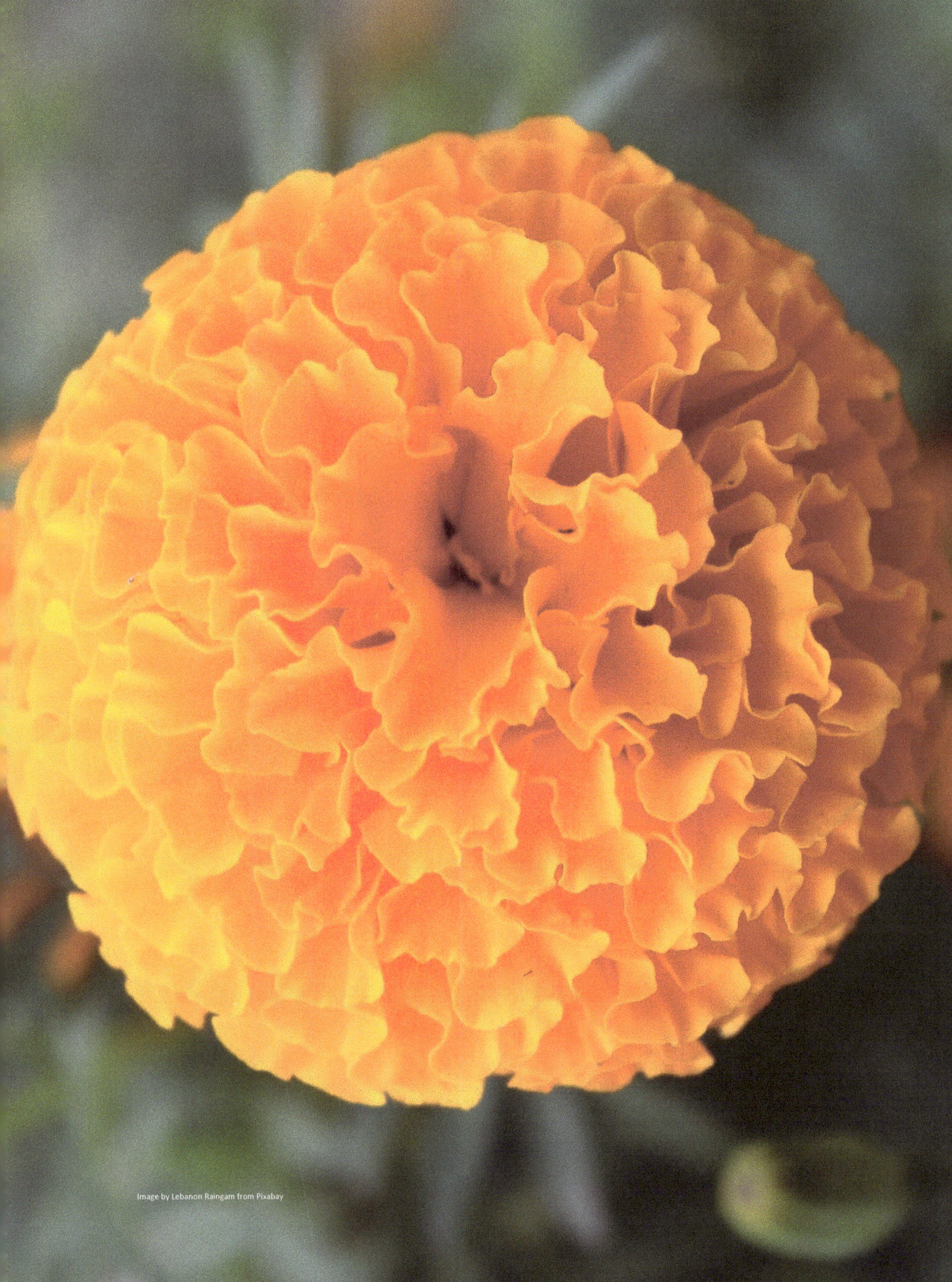
Image by Lebanon Raingam from Pixabay

Marigold - Tagetes erecta

Marigold is a popular flower and sought after when in bloom all around the world. There are approximately fifty species of Marigold, however the three types of Marigold of interest here are the American variety Tagetes erecta, which has larger flowers than the French Marigold Tagetes patula, and Mexican tarragon Tagetes lucida once again from South America. For some strange reason T. erecta is also known as African Marigold, however, it is native to Mexico and South America and not Africa. At any rate, they are the same variety.

Marigold has long been used in herbal medicines throughout its natural range. The north American Indians used the flower and leaves as a skin wash for infections and fungal conditions. The Aztecs used the flowers for eye infections. In Brazil, it is used for vermifuge (worms), inflammation and joint pain. In Mexico, it is used as a carminative and diuretic. Therefore, there are a wide range of traditional uses and claims associated with Marigold. Its use as an antibiotic and antiseptic has also been validated in clinical research, as well as its use as an antioxidant. It showed better results when compared to vitamin C (ascorbic acid). Due to the high levels of beta carotenoids in the flowers, science has shown the extract to be useful for improving eyesight. Interestingly the flowers may be added to salads as it has been shown to be non-toxic.

Marigolds have been adopted throughout the world and integrated into the herbal lore and cultures of many nations. In India, it is considered a holy flower and used to garland holy men, statues, and temples. In Ukraine the flower is a symbol of the nation. In its native range, the flower is associated with death and the departed. As a result, the flower is used almost exclusively for the national Day of the Dead and is commonly planted in cemeteries throughout the Southern Americas. The Aztecs reportedly used the flowers as a dried powder that was blown into the faces of those about to be sacrificed because it was believed to relax them and make the victims more pliant and happier about their impending deaths. If a plant can make you happy about that, then it is definitely a flower to use in depression.

Claims that the extract derived from the leaves and flowers have antidepressant and anticonvulsant actions have also been substantiated in clinical research. It is believed that the plant extract works on the serotonin levels in the body and therefore elevates these hormones. The investigation into the Mexican claims that the use of the flowers as a tisane and also a tincture supported the anxiolytic (anti-anxiety) and sedative claims. Additional research has been conducted on the antidepressant actions of the plant and have found that it is not dose-dependent, and that higher doses had sedative actions. As a result, care should be taken if you wish to stay alert when using the plant.

The essential oil made from the flowers and the leaves is sold commercially, however, care should be taken when buying it from manufacturers with less than ideal reputations as it may be adulterated with non-essential base oils. Tagetes erecta may be used as either a tisane, tincture, or oil.

[1] P. Gupta and N. Vasudeva, "A Potential Ornamental Plant Drug," Hamdard Med., vol. 55, no. 1, pp. 45–59, 2012.

[2] L. J. Shetty, F. M. Sakr, K. Al-Obaidy, M. J. Patel, and H. Shareef, "A brief review on medicinal plant Tagetes erecta Linn," J. Appl. Pharm. Sci., vol. 5, no. Suppl 3, pp. 091–095, 2015.

[3] B. Salehi et al., Tagetes spp. Essential oils and other extracts: Chemical characterization and biological activity, vol. 23, no. 11. 2018.

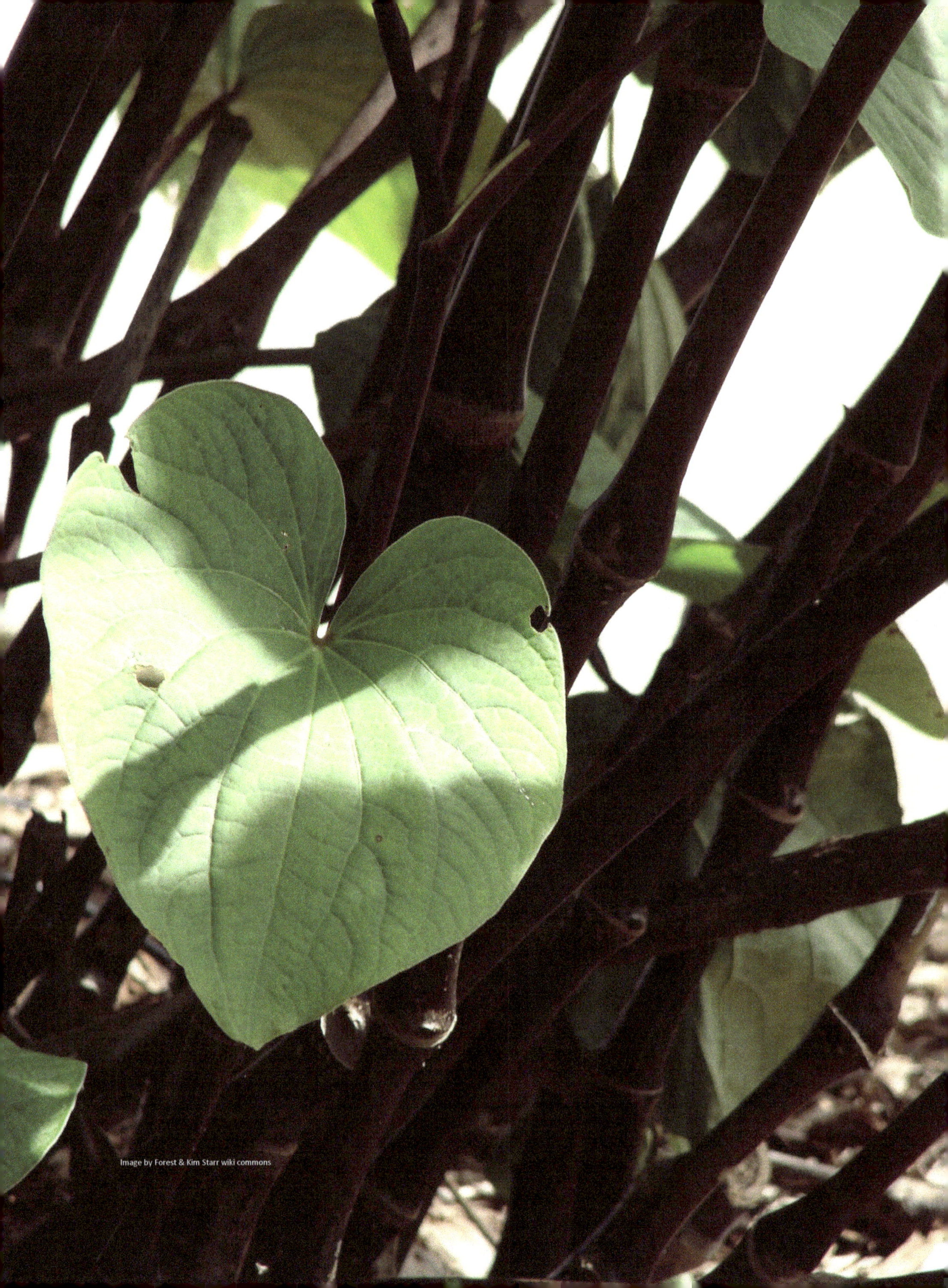
Image by Forest & Kim Starr wiki commons

Kava - Piper methysticum

Throughout the islands of the Pacific Ocean, the roots of Piper methysticum have been used for centuries as both a ceremonial drink and an everyday social drink. It is known throughout the region by many names such as yaqona, kava, waka, ava, awa, seka, sekau and melok. In many island nations, such as Fiji, it is consumed in groups of people around a large wooden bowl known as a tanoa from which it is poured into a half coconut shell, known as bilo, which is then passed around the group.

There has been much controversy associated with Kava in the early part of this century as it was claimed to damage liver tissue over time. These claims have been reversed, and various clinical trials have failed to substantiate the reported risks. Of all the information available, perhaps the most reliable is the anecdotal evidence that liver disease is relatively unknown in the Pacific Islands where it has been in use for thousands of years. There is one apparent side effect from overuse of the herb, and this is evident by the skin becoming dry and flaky, which is commonly called 'kani-kani' in the Fijian language. This condition clears when the use of Kava is reduced or stopped. It is prudent that pregnant women should not use Kava as it has been associated with babies being underweight. In light of the controversy surrounding the use of Kava and possible side effects, it is the only herb studied that should be used in an aqueous (water-based) manner as most of the reported negative cases have been from extracts made with acetone or methanol. The traditional method of preparing the herb is soaking the powdered root in cold water, however a much better and more palatable approach is making a tea from the desiccated roots.

Kava has been recognised as being highly effective in treating anxiety and depression, amongst other health claims such as hypertension. The active compounds in Piper methysticum are known as kavalactones. These are kavain, desmethoxyyangonin and yangonin, and they are higher in the roots than in the stems and leaves, with dihydrokavain, methysticin, and dihydromethysticin being present.

Clinical studies have shown that whilst Kava is an effective anti-anxiety and antidepressant, it also acts as a muscle relaxant and sedative. Therefore, it may not be the best choice if you need to be active and alert.

In a study carried out in Queensland Australia in 2009, it was shown that the aqueous extract of Kava displayed a significant reduction in anxiety and depression in 60 adult volunteers over one month.

The World Health Organisation (WHO) has included Kava in its library of herbal monographs, and supports the use of the herb for insomnia, anxiety, central nervous system support, spasm, convulsions and pain management. In the report it was stated that a study of 4049 people who used Kava over a 7 week period only 1.5% showed any adverse effects from the herb and the most common side effect was gastrointestinal upset.

[1] M. F. D. Amorim et al., "The controvertible role of kava (Piper methysticum G. Foster) an anxiolytic herb, on toxic hepatitis," Brazilian J. Pharmacogn., vol. 17, no. 3, pp. 448–454, 2007.

[2] G. Lee and H. Bae, "Therapeutic effects of phytochemicals and medicinal herbs on depression," Biomed Res. Int., vol. 2017, 2017.

[3] European Medicines Agency (EMA), "Public statement on Piper methysticum G. Forst., rhizoma," vol. 44, no. November, 2016.

[4] L. Greek, P. Islands, and P. Ocean, "Kava."

You can't hide from yourself

"Every time I have tried to run from myself, I have found myself standing on the next crossing, ahead of me"

Sukant Ratnaka

Pending on which paper or person you rely on for information it is estimated that approximately 300 million people are currently suffering from depression. Needless to say, this number is, in all reality, a vast underestimation.

More and more research is being undertaken to find why depression and anxiety are the bed rock of many other psychological problems. Today it is now considered obvious that drug and substance abuse, compulsive eating, alcoholism, anorexia, hypersexuality or compulsive behaviours are some of the negative psychological states that have at their core a depressed person. As a result, to help these people at some stage they all have to be introduced to something that they fear the most....which is of course themselves.

Life has all manner of facets within its majestic weave and loom. Some good, many plain boring, a few wonderful and many threads are simply full of pain. Naturally, it is logical for us to avoid pain and in most cases, as this would appear as very sound common sense, yet there are many examples that this avoidance does not cure the cause of the pain but actually feeds it quietly in the background making it stronger until the day it will not remain hidden or ignored any longer.

Experience over time will educate us as to a vast array of things that may hurt us. We know that electricity is a modern-day wonder, even though it can kill us. Therefore, we learn how to cope with the negative or dangerous aspects of it in our lives. In research from 1993 by Moos, R.H. and Schaefer, J.A. titled *"Coping Resources and Processes: Current Concepts and Measures"* is an early scientific attempt at understanding how we process or avoid emotional trauma or negative emotions. The authors stated that coping processes can have a focus that is based on either approaching or avoiding the problem and a method that is primarily either cognitive or behavioural, making up four basic types of coping strategies: cognitive approach, behavioural approach, cognitive avoidance, and behavioural avoidance. Put in plain terms we can either use our intelligence to process and thereby control our reactions or simply change our behaviour i.e., stop smoking. Conversely, we can avoid these traumas and emotions intellectually by thinking about other things or develop a behaviour that helps us avoid negative thoughts such as the obsessive-compulsive disorder (OCD) of constantly cleaning our surroundings. This last point was the finding from a 2016 study that found cleaning was the most popular activity of people experiencing OCD (72%). However, we are making the mistake of thinking that the behaviours or thoughts that we employ, in order to avoid depression, are all negative or possibly psychologically harmful and this is a completely imbalanced view. What is normal for one person may be abnormal for another. Let's look at the person who spends several hours in their local gym every day, yes, they may have the body of a god or goddess, but their quality of life may be awful. In the majority of cases this devotion to the gym can be found to be a healthy and balanced choice yet there is another common personality type engaged in this activity and that is the person who has image issues and identity insecurities.

Regardless, we will not rest there as many other examples of avoidance can be found and intellectually dissected. Continuous travel, overworking, binge movie watching, voracious book reading, hypochondria (fascination with illnesses and disease) may all be driven as ways of avoiding depression. In a twist we begin to realise that some of our greatest discoveries or achievements, in our history have a depressed person to thank. They in turn can thank their depression.

So, the question we all have to ask ourselves, regardless of whether you are depressed or not, is "Are my thoughts or behaviours hiding something about myself that I do not wish to face?". When considering this please keep in mind that the people in asylums who think that they are perfectly sane are usually the patients. In our minds, time and space are irrelevant as we can imagine the past present and future and fit in concepts of the universe. Hence, our internal psychological environments are vast, and we can hide all manner of dark and painful landscapes within it. Nearly all of us have a few simple regrets about events in our past. The "I wish I did that differently!" is almost universal. However, the ideology that "Oh, I'm not that interesting let's talk about someone else!" may be the clue to low self-esteem or value and a pre curser to a realm of depression.

Now we know that to follow this line of questioning it would be very easy to arrive at the statement that basically everyone on the planet is depressed! Obviously, this cannot be true. Remember all those morons! There are actually a lot of happy people out there in the world! We are discussing, however, all the people who are very very good at avoiding themselves and their own emptiness. Any discussion on depression would only be half complete if it did not address those in denial or avoiding themselves.

There are those who are actually too busy to be depressed. Those people who are holding everything together and sacrificing themselves for the good of others. The single parent. The bread winner working three jobs. The carer taking care of the vulnerable and infirm. Even if some of these people do have an underlying issue with anxiety and depression the last thing they would or even could do is take the time out to attempt reconnecting with their own desires and needs. The outcome if they tried this has a high probability of being disastrous and their worlds would fall apart. Rather, the best strategy they could use is to initially recognize that they may have underlying issues such as depression. Then the acceptance that at this time in their lives they do not have the luxury or resources to tackle these challenges and then mentally prepare for the time when they do have the time. A similarity would be the person who after working incredibly hard, for months on end, finally gets to go on the holiday they have been dreaming about only to fall sick on the second day and spend the next two weeks in bed. After putting their bodies through all that stress in their jobs once they finally relax their bodies collapse and enter a state of repair. It is the same for those who are too busy to be depressed. These people are not denying or avoiding they simply can't afford the luxury of being depressed which is a uniquely strange statement.

Those people who are not aware that they are running away from themselves are the ones most at risk of slipping into major depression. This is largely due to the fact that because of their denial they do not begin to develop any coping mechanisms. They are completely unprepared when the depressive episodes begin and as a result experience them far worse than a person who has been dealing with depression as an everyday occurrence.

The reality is that no one is able to run away from depression, it is already packed in your luggage before you even get to the door. The only thing avoidance is guaranteed to do is make matters worse when the time finally comes and there is no more emotional energy to keep the demons away.

Dealing with depression has the critical first step of admitting to it. You might be able to hide from yourself for a while but never from an eager and determined canine nose that will come sniffing for you when you are hiding silently in some hallway cupboard.

[1] M. M. Dar, T. Ahmad Bhat, S. Maqbool, M. A. Paul, and R. Bhat, "Hospital Based Study of Depression among OCD Patients," *Int. J. Contemp. Med. Res.*, vol. 3, no. 11, pp. 2454–7379, 2016.

[2] E. Altintaş and N. Taşkintuna, "Factors associated with depression in obsessive-compulsive disorder: A cross-sectional study," *Noropsikiyatri Ars.*, vol. 52, no. 4, pp. 346–353, 2015.

[3] J. W. Kanter, A. M. Busch, C. E. Weeks, and S. J. Landes, "The nature of clinical depression: Symptoms, syndromes, and behavior analysis," *Behav. Anal.*, vol. 31, no. 1, pp. 1–21, 2008.

[4] J. P. Carvalho, "Avoidance and Depression : Evidence for Reinforcement as a Mediating Factor," 2011.

[5] J. W. Kanter, D. E. Baruch, and S. T. Gaynor, "Acceptance and commitment therapy and behavioral activation for the treatment of depression: Description and comparison," *Behav. Anal.*, vol. 29, no. 2, pp. 161–185, 2006.

[6] J. W. Kanter, L. C. Rusch, A. M. Busch, and S. K. Sedivy, "Validation of the behavioral activation for depression scale (BADS) in a community sample with elevated depressive symptoms," *J. Psychopathol. Behav. Assess.*, vol. 31, no. 1, pp. 36–42, 2009.

[7] I. Schreiner and J. P. Malcolm, "The benefits of mindfulness meditation: Changes in emotional states of depression, anxiety, and stress," *Behav. Chang.*, vol. 25, no. 3, pp. 156–168, 2008.

[8] R. J. McNally, P. Mair, B. L. Mugno, and B. C. Riemann, "Co-morbid obsessive-compulsive disorder and depression: A Bayesian network approach," *Psychol. Med.*, vol. 47, no. 7, pp. 1204–1214, 2017.

[9] M. E. Sorbero *et al.*, "Meditation for depression a systematic review of mindfulness-based cognitive therapy for major depressive disorder," *Natl. Def. Res. Inst.*, no. October, pp. 1–179, 2015.

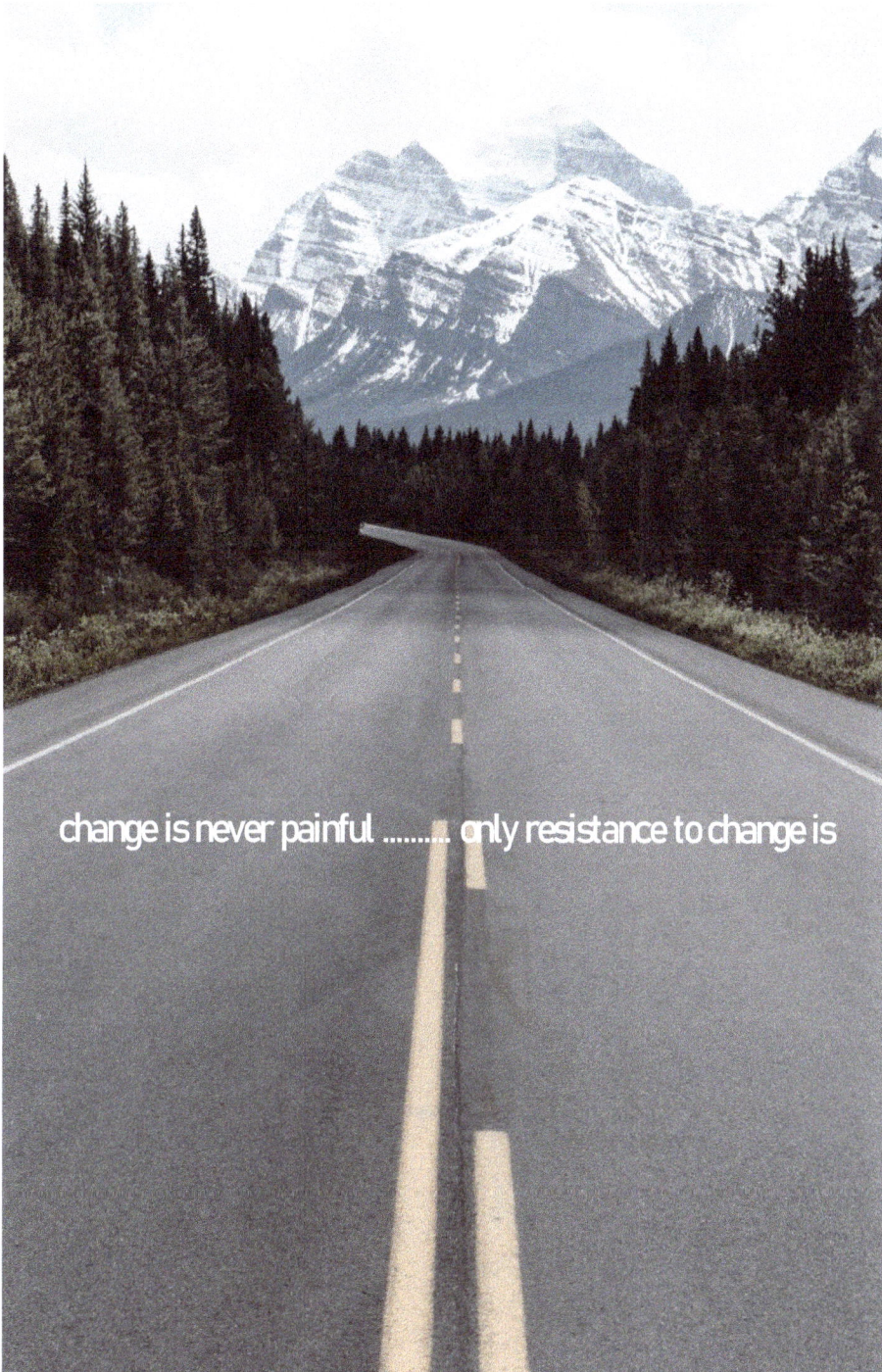

change is never painful .... only resistance to change is

Image by Public Co from Pixabay

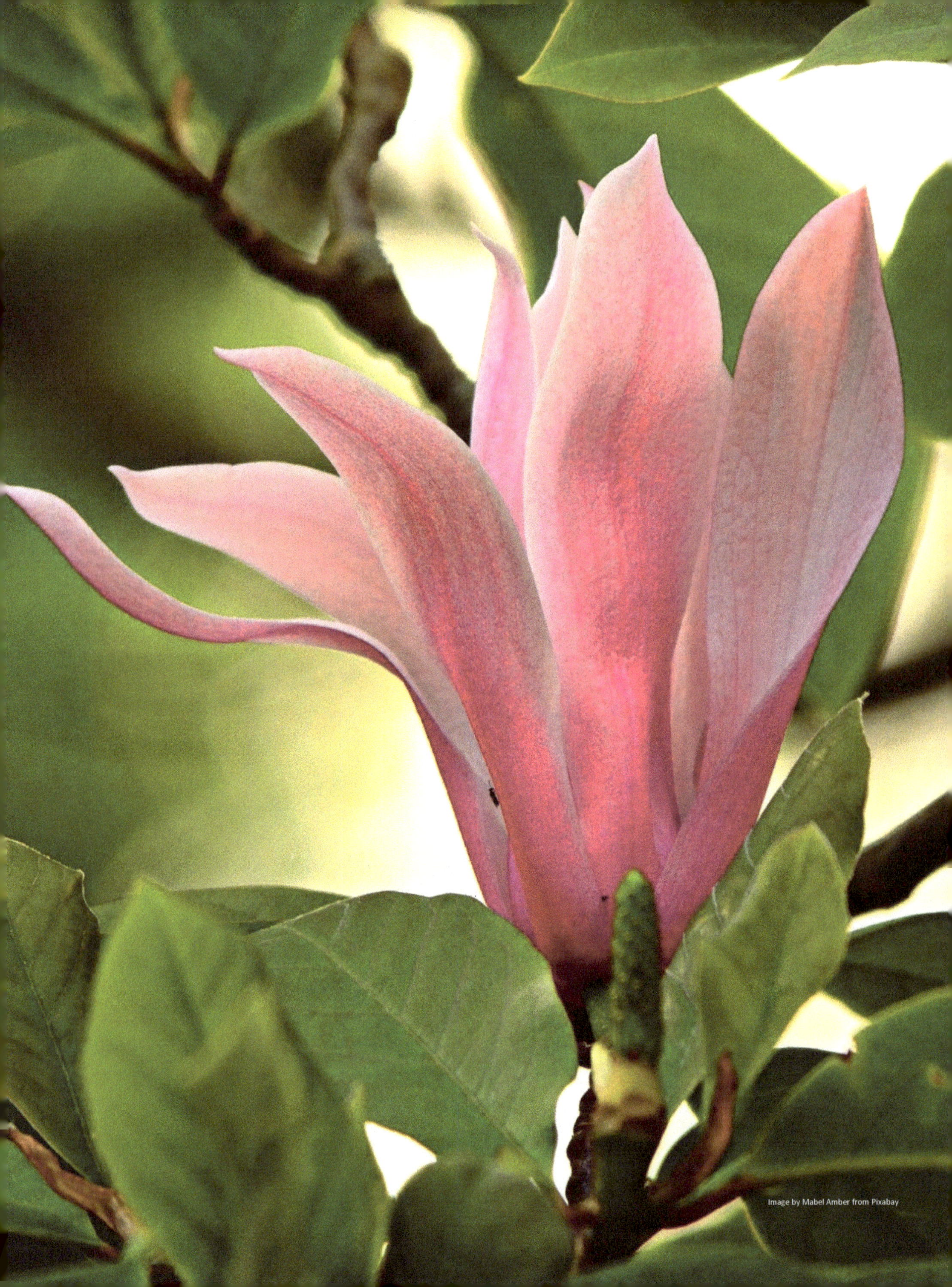
Image by Mabel Amber from Pixabay

Magnolia - Magnolia

The members of the Magnolia family are renowned for their beautiful flowers, and it has made them a favourite for gardens and city parks. The family of this tree has approximately 350 members and is named after the French botanist Pierre Magnol. It has been reported that the first identified Magnolia tree was located in the Caribbean, however since then it has been found that the tree and its brethren are spread in South East Asia, North and South America as well as the Caribbean region. Magnolias are thought to belong to a small group of trees considered to be living fossils. It's probable that the shifting continents over time have separated populations of the trees, due to which isolated groups grew unique attributes and differences, thereby creating the different members of the Magnolia family. The flowers of the trees have supposedly adapted for insects rather than bees to pollinate them. This is thought to be clear evidence that the trees existed in prehistory well before bees had evolved and therefore had to rely on the large prehistoric beetles to do the work for them. Other members of this 'living fossil' group are the Wollemi Pine and Ginkgo Biloba.

The use of Magnolia in traditional health systems has occurred throughout Asia especially Japan and China, and it could also be assumed the North American species such as M. grandiflora would have also been used by the indigenous people of South-eastern United States. In China, the bark of the tree is used for the treatment of various ailments and is known by the name 'houpo'.

Research has shown the trees are rich in compounds that are slowly being unlocked by science as to their health benefits and applications. Two of these compounds that are unique to the Magnolia family are honokiol and magnolol. It is believed that these two compounds are responsible for the antidepressant actions of the bark extract. Research from 2019 showed that honokiol reduced inflammatory conditions in the body, especially in the central nervous system.

Within the same study, it was noted that the use of magnolia extracts reduced the levels of 'quinolinic acid' in the brain. This acid is a by-product of certain brain functions and has been associated with psychotic conditions and neurodegenerative processes of brain tissue. Also, there was an additional reduction in free calcium levels in the brain tissue, thereby reducing calcium overload. As a result, the use of Magnolia not only relieves depression and anxiety, but is also a tonic for brain function and health. In a research study from the United Kingdom (2017) into the possible misuse of Magnolia, it was found that there is little evidence that Magnolia is dangerous in any singular form. It was this review paper that clarified that Magnolia compounds interact with the CB1 and CB2 receptors in the body. These receptors are also sensitive to cannabis.

Other effects associated with Magnolia are improved sleep, lowered anxiety, weight loss, reduced bowel inflammation and possible cancer management properties.

[1] B. Zhang et al., "Antidepressant-like effect and mechanism of action of honokiol on the mouse lipopolysaccharide (LPS) depression model," Molecules, vol. 24, no. 11, pp. 1–17, 2019.

[2] M. Poivre and P. Duez, "Biological activity and toxicity of the Chinese herb Magnolia officinalis Rehder & E. Wilson (Houpo) and its constituents," J. Zhejiang Univ. Sci. B, vol. 18, no. 3, pp. 194–214, 2017.

[3] J. You et al., "후박의 항우울 효과에 대한 실험적 연구," vol. 34, no. 3, pp. 256–266, 2013.

[4] F. Schifano, V. Guarino, D. G. Papanti, J. Baccarin, L. Orsolini, and J. M. Corkery, "Is there a potential of misuse for Magnolia officinalis compounds/metabolites?," Hum. Psychopharmacol., vol. 32, no. 3, pp. 1–7, 2017.

[5] S. M. Talbott, J. A. Talbott, and M. Pugh, "Effect of Magnolia officinalis and Phellodendron amurense (Relora®) on cortisol and psychological mood state in moderately stressed subjects," J. Int. Soc. Sports Nutr., vol. 10, no. 1, p. 1, 2013.

[6] S. B, "Antidepressants: Mechanism of Action, Toxicity and Possible Amelioration," J. Appl. Biotechnol. Bioeng., vol. 3, no. 5, pp. 437–448, 2017.

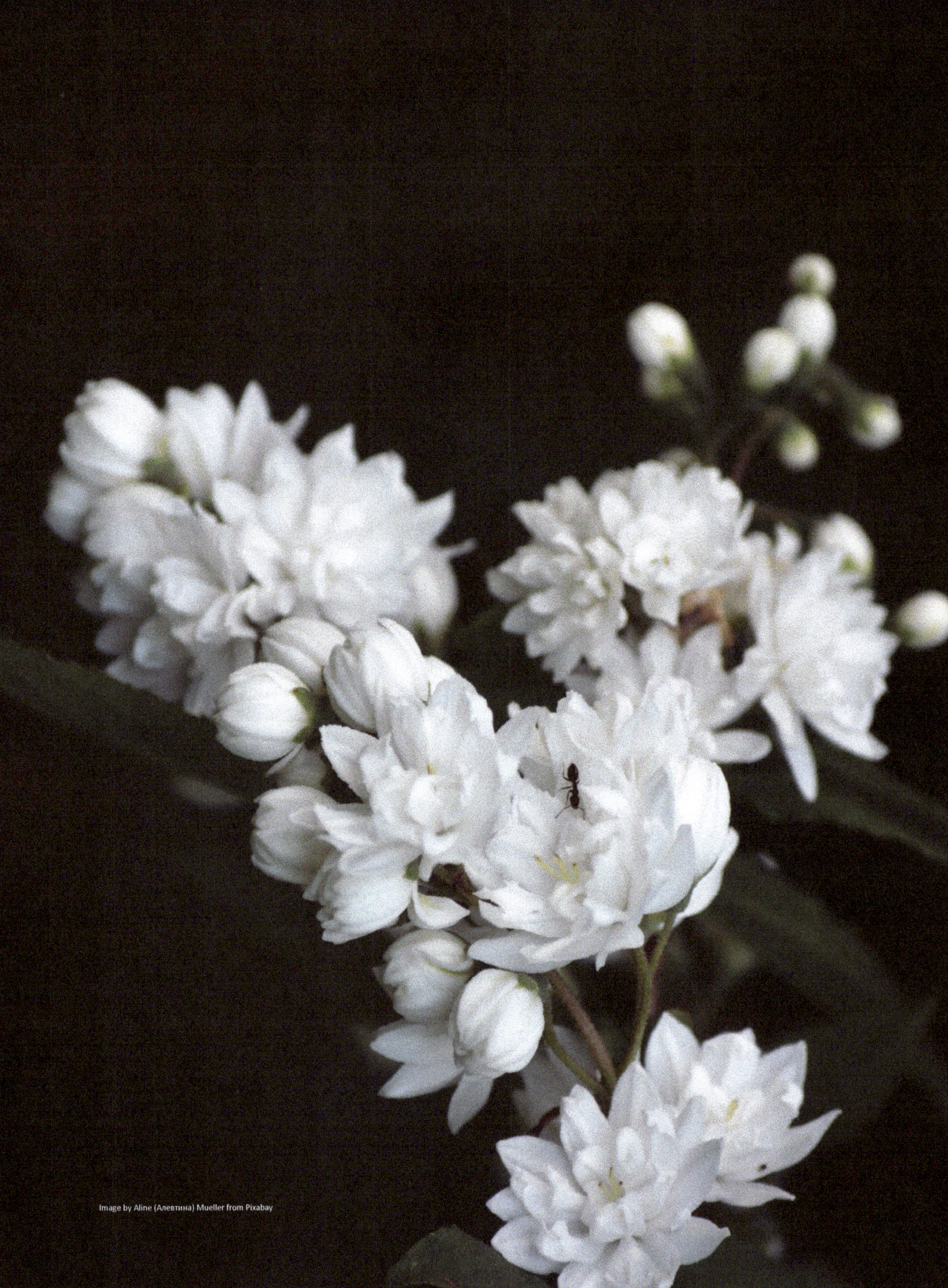

Image by Aline (Алевтина) Mueller from Pixabay

Arabian Jasmine - Jasminum sambac

Jasmine has been used for hundreds of years for a wide range of health conditions such as mouth infections, weakness of sight, ulcers, insanity, leprosy, skin disorders, analgesic, anti-inflammatory, antidepressant, antiseptic, aphrodisiac, calmative, cytotoxic and expectorant. Whilst some of these claims have not been supported by scientific research, the antidepressant actions of the flowers and leaves have. The plant originates from South East Asia, yet due to the unique aroma or perfume of the flowers it is now grown throughout the world. The flowers are primarily associated with Buddhism, are the national flower of the Philippines, and are used in the manufacture of Jasmine tea.

In a research paper from 2014 it was found that doses of the leaf extract are at levels of between 250 mg/kg and 500 mg/kg body weight. The results from this research showed that the higher dose of 500 mg had similar therapeutic effects as that of the standard drug imipramine in the alleviation of depression. The plant has various chemical compounds, some of which are sambacin, jasminum, sambacoside A, sambacolignoside, quercetin, isoquercetin, rutin, kaempferol, ursolic acid, linalool, phenyl methanol, and glucoside-sambacoside. As with a great deal of research into plant medicines, the researchers here sought to understand if the plant had any toxicity. They found that doses up to 2000 mg/kg were considered safe. The conclusion from this research was that the leaf extract elevated both serotonin and dopamine monoamines but not norepinephrine.

Additional research, this time from Iraq in 2018, discussed various medical applications of the oil from the flowers of the Jasmine plant. The anti-inflammatory actions of the oil were shown to be significant and would aid in the reduction of inflammatory conditions that may exacerbate depression and anxiety. It was found by the researchers of this paper that merely the smell of Jasmine tea had a measurable effect on the reduction of stress and anxiety. It was also shown that test volunteers experienced reduced heart rates and a lowering of overall blood pressure. This paper from Iraq also supported the use of the oil, flowers, and leaves from the plant in the treatment of depression and anxiety.

Going back to 2012, an article that appeared in the "International Research Journal of Pharmaceutical and Applied Sciences" compared the antidepressant actions of Jasmine oil against other essential oils such as sandalwood, agarwood, eucalyptus and lemon oils and found that Jasmine oil was more effective. Much of the scientific literature on the use of Jasmine in the treatment of depression support its use. A paper (below) from 2013 is another such example.

[1] Sabharwal, "Jasminum Sambac Linn (Motia): a Review," Int. J. Pharm. Res. Bio-Science, vol. 2, no. 5, pp. 108–130, 2013.

[2] T. K. Lim and T. K. Lim, "Jasminum sambac," Edible Med. Non Med. Plants, pp. 529–540, 2014.

[3] A. E. Al-snafi, "Pharmacological And Therapeutic Effects Of Jasminum Sambac - A Review," Indo Am. J. Pfharmaceutical Sci., vol. 05, no. 03, pp. 1766–1778, 2018.

[4] V. Anusha, S. Asma, K. Ratnakumari, and N. Govindamma, "Int . Res J Pharm . App Sci ., 2012 ; 2 (3): 9-12 Research Article Anti-depressant activity of some aroma oils on mice," vol. 2, no. Iii, pp. 9–12, 2012.

[5] I. Of and I. Of, "Antidepressant Like Effects of Jasminum Sambac – Investigation of Involvement of Monoaminergic System," vol. 3, no. 6, pp. 755–770, 2014.

Metaphorical suicide

"Nobody can go back and start a new beginning.
But anyone can start today and make a new ending"

Maria Robinson

More than 800,000 people die annually because of suicide, which is the second leading cause of death among people in the age group of 15-29 years.

Suicide is simply the act of taking one's own life in any method, no matter whether it is aided or unaided. This may appear a confusing statement until we consider euthanasia or voluntary assisted dying for those with excruciating terminal illnesses. The act is quite simply the act. The reasoning behind doing such act is where I focus the debate. No discussion on depression can survive scrutiny without at least touching on this topic. Labelled a sin and a crime, the act of taking one's own life has been the subject of romantic loathing and onto the act of absolute self-indulgence. As such, a great deal of useless rational baggage has accumulated around the discussion that makes it harder to dissect its necessary parts, or, if you like, to conduct a beneficial autopsy on the topic. Dark humour is a necessary spice when sitting down to an intellectual meal such as this one.

Regardless of the statistics or reports you may have read, it would be fair to say that many of them are wrong as suicide pervades all age groups and demographics. We simply don't see it the same way. When the body of an old and lonely woman is found several days after her death in her home full of memories and faded colours, we simply rush to state 'natural causes'. Yet, a handsome son whose body is being carefully removed, bit by gruesome bit, under the midnight floodlights over railway tracks we rush to pronounce 'youth suicide' and belabour the tragedy of it. Both are tragedies yet depending on your point of view it may appear that the lonely forgotten woman in her years of isolation discarded by society may be all the more poignant rather than the 'selfish' young man who suffered for a few months, and by one quick and desperate act has traumatised rescue teams, train drivers and the boy's confused family. It is at this point that you can hear the rising roar of indignant youth, social workers, therapists, and families of those carrying scars left on the living, after suicide tore their families apart. Screaming indignation against such callous words. All we can do when entering a minefield of emotions and pain is to either tread so lightly that our words have no impact or gleefully rampage with equal emotion and commitment across it watching the cathartic explosions occur. When such a debate starts to reach a point like this one is, the predominant rebuke is "How would you know of my pain?", or "How can you be so uncaring?", or equally "You have no idea!", and to which, I will now switch to the 'first-person, and I calmly say "Oh, yes I do." Because suicide is to a large part a hidden and unspoken facet of many people's lives, there are more witnesses and survivors than you could possibly imagine. I am merely one such survivor.

The aim here on this page is not to talk with the therapist or remaining family member but to talk directly to you, the person considering suicide. The person considering a permanent solution to a short-term problem. In order to get access to the mind and inner workings of such a person they will only consider a counter point of view when the point of view is coming from someone who has also experienced, whilst not the same, then the same intensity of sorrow and pain. Therefore, allow me a moment to share my vulnerability, shame and despair when I was a young man.

I will not share the graphic details but rather the type. I was the type who never discussed my thoughts with others. Never did I threaten suicide to another person. Never did I seek help. I was one of those people who from one day to the next arrived dead. I didn't fear death but rather yearned for it. I was methodical in my execution. Calm in my logic and reasoning. I remember the afternoon after I had ingested in excess of 120 sleeping pills as some of the most tranquil hours in my life at that young naive age. I single-mindedly and desperately wanted my situation to end. It was only by a quirk of timing that I was found and rushed to the ER. One memory that stayed with me over 40 years later is opening my eyes to stare at an industrial hospital ceiling, allowing the slow and depressing realisation that I was still alive, and thinking that not only had I failed at my life, but I had also failed in ending it. That level of depression is an entirely new low and I had found that the house of Depression had a hidden basement in it, waiting just for me. There was no joy, no thankfulness at finding myself alive. Yet years later, I breathe a sigh of relief that I have found joy, and on most days I thank my lucky stars that I am still alive. As a result, please excuse me for being blunt, I reiterate that suicide is the most selfish and self-indulgent act a person can undertake. However, there are exceptions.

One such exception is the still current debate surrounding euthanasia or voluntary assisted dying for the terminally ill. Such illnesses left to transpire on their natural course of the disease, wracking the body of the sufferer and will in the end result in death. Medicine, impotent to cure or alleviate, has only the option of standing to one side. Medicine in the form of a poison however provides the final medication. The financial destruction, the youthful sacrifice of children in caring for the sick elders and the emotional pain of loved ones as they can only watch in anger and despair does not even take into account the sufferer's pain, shame and loss of dignity. To allow such a person afflicted by such cruelty the one act, the one last decision to not be a sufferer, but to have some semblance of power would be a kindness, not a crime. Counter to this is the person or groups who demand that the individual suffering from such illness is to endure every last second of its impact until such a time as the last sodden putrid breath has had its way with their bodies. These people who deny a death of dignity would in many people's minds be committing a heinous crime akin to a malignant and sadistic murder.

From here we can discuss other such potential exceptions, needless to say, the colours become greyer and the boundaries vaguer. I am sure we can all sympathise with a person undergoing daily abuses of the most horrific kind, such as that experienced by the young Yazidi girls enslaved by the Islamic State. Would you be strong enough to endure month after month of degradation not knowing how many of your family members had been murdered or suffering the same as you? Or would you, like many of these women, prefer to take the only door open to them. The door called suicide.

Then we come again to the lonely woman in her house of memories and faded colours. Whilst her suicide might be more understandable and easier to accept because we can justify the act as she had no one left to hurt. No one would miss her. No one would see the waste of youth, beauty and potential. Her suicide is and will always be carried out with self-pity and self-indulgence at the forefront of the decision. She felt lonely. She felt unloved. She felt useless and perhaps other dark feelings. Yet taking her own life ten years before the alcohol and cigarettes could do their jobs is still a waste. Here we come to the term Metaphysical Suicide. The act of ending a life begs us to ask what is a Life? Is it defined by the continual beating of a heart or is it also the entirety of things; the house, the job, the friends or lack of them? If it is the entirety of things, then ending a life might not necessarily be plunging that dagger into your breast. It might not be that early morning leap from that cliff. It might not be that toxic cocktail of pharmaceuticals mixed with rum. It may simply be the closing of the front door and a quietly spoken "Fuck you!" as you kill your present, and soon to be past life while walking into a new one yet to be built. In essence, carrying out a Metaphysical Suicide.

In many countries, this is occurring every day and is described as 'runaways' or 'disappearances'. The caring family man who leaves to purchase that missing bottle of milk for the children's meal only to not return as he just kept on going. Never touching the bank account or credit card again. Not taking to the family car. Not contacting friends or associates. The daughter who, one morning, does not come to breakfast. The work associate who simply stops coming to work. We can only guess as to what they have run away from. What demons in their minds? What abuse they can no longer tolerate. They simply cease to exist except in the memories of those they have left behind. In some ways, these Disappearances may be more painful due to the doubt of whether they had been a victim of foul play. They may be trapped in some basement or worse. A simple note left to be found days later may offer some comfort to those left behind and this may be far preferable to finding a dead body after a traditional suicide. In Japan, an entire section of the society is known as the 'johatsu' or 'evaporated people'. In this country, there are even agents who can help you disappear known as 'yonige-ya' which translates as 'fly by night shops.'

Up until this point we have engaged in a high level and unemotional discussion on the topic, yet depression and its influence on the mind of the sufferer is a difficult maze to unravel. Depression is a debilitating health condition that may be considered predominantly intellectual, as such that the logic of the sufferer is skewed toward self-harm. This may express itself merely by isolating yourself from the support of others or all the way across the spectrum to the serious consideration of death being preferable to a life of depression. We must keep in mind that suicide is at the extreme end of a spectrum of thought and behaviour. It resides at the most extreme dark edge of depression, and the sufferer must realise that all their other thoughts, no matter how logical and or balanced they seem, are completely out of balance and not logical in the slightest. As a result, should you or anyone else you may know consider suicide it is a sure sign that you are in no state to make any decisions at all, other than coffee + doughnut/ repeat, until better.

[1] D. A. Rund and R. V. Saveanu, 'Depression and suicide,' Emerg. Med. Secrets, vol. 124, no. 1, pp. 663–669, 2011.

[2] M. Nakao and T. Takeuchi, 'The suicide epidemic in Japan and strategies of depression screening for its prevention.,' Bull. World Health Organ., vol. 84, no. 6, pp. 492–493, 2006.

[3] Y. Conwell, 'Depression as a 'cause' of late life suicide.,' Crisis, vol. 13, no. 2, pp. 55–56, 1992.

[4] J. Kitanaka, 'Depression in Japan: Psychiatric cures for a society in distress,' Depress. Japan Psychiatr. Cures a Soc. Distress, no. April, pp. 1–243, 2011.

[5] N. Izadinia, M. Amiri, R. G. Jahromi, and S. Hamidi, 'A study of relationship between suicidal ideas, depression, anxiety, resiliency, daily stresses and mental health among Tehran university students,' Procedia - Soc. Behav. Sci., vol. 5, pp. 1615–1619, 2010.

,

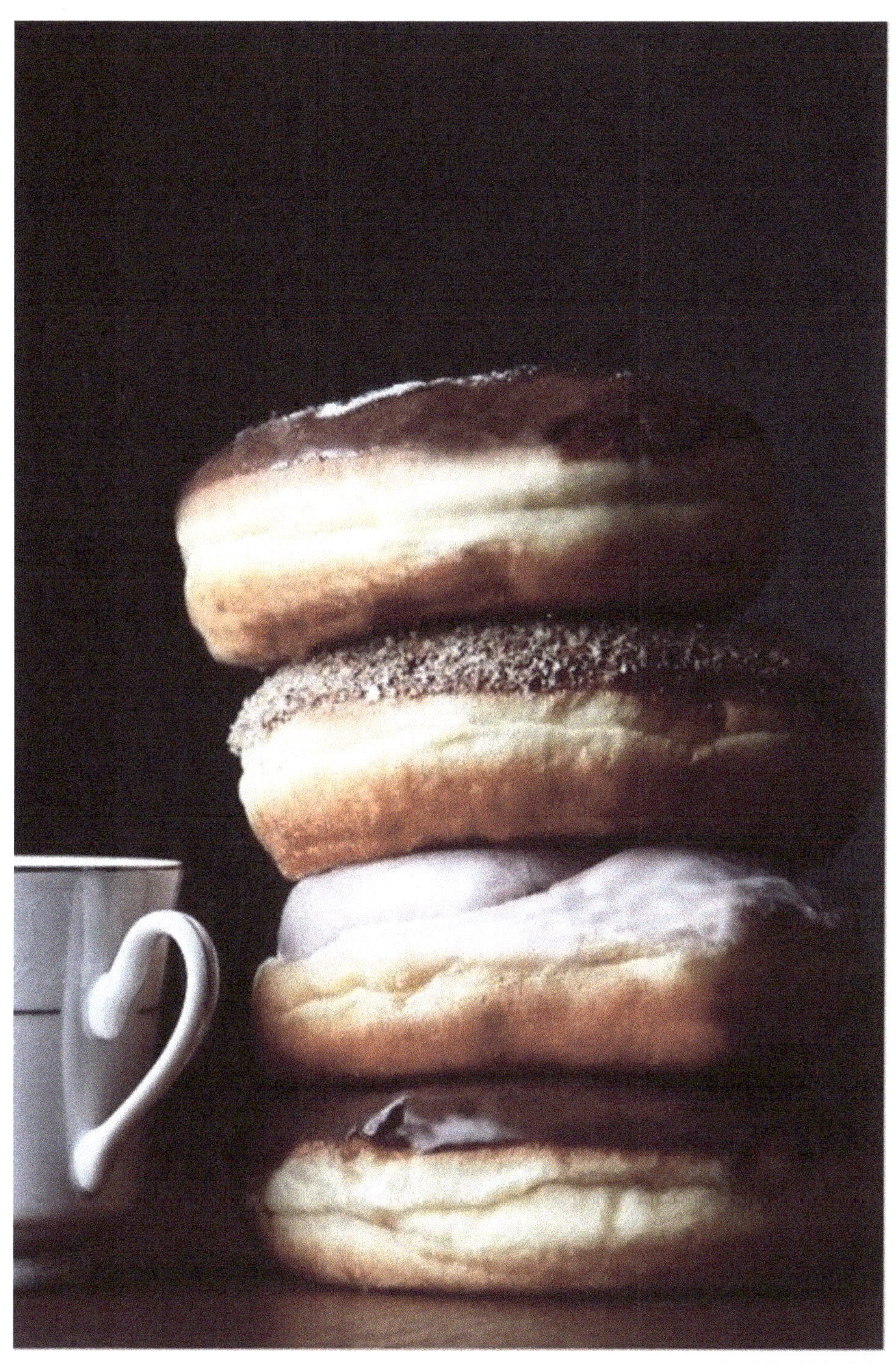

Image by Zitouniatis from Pixabay

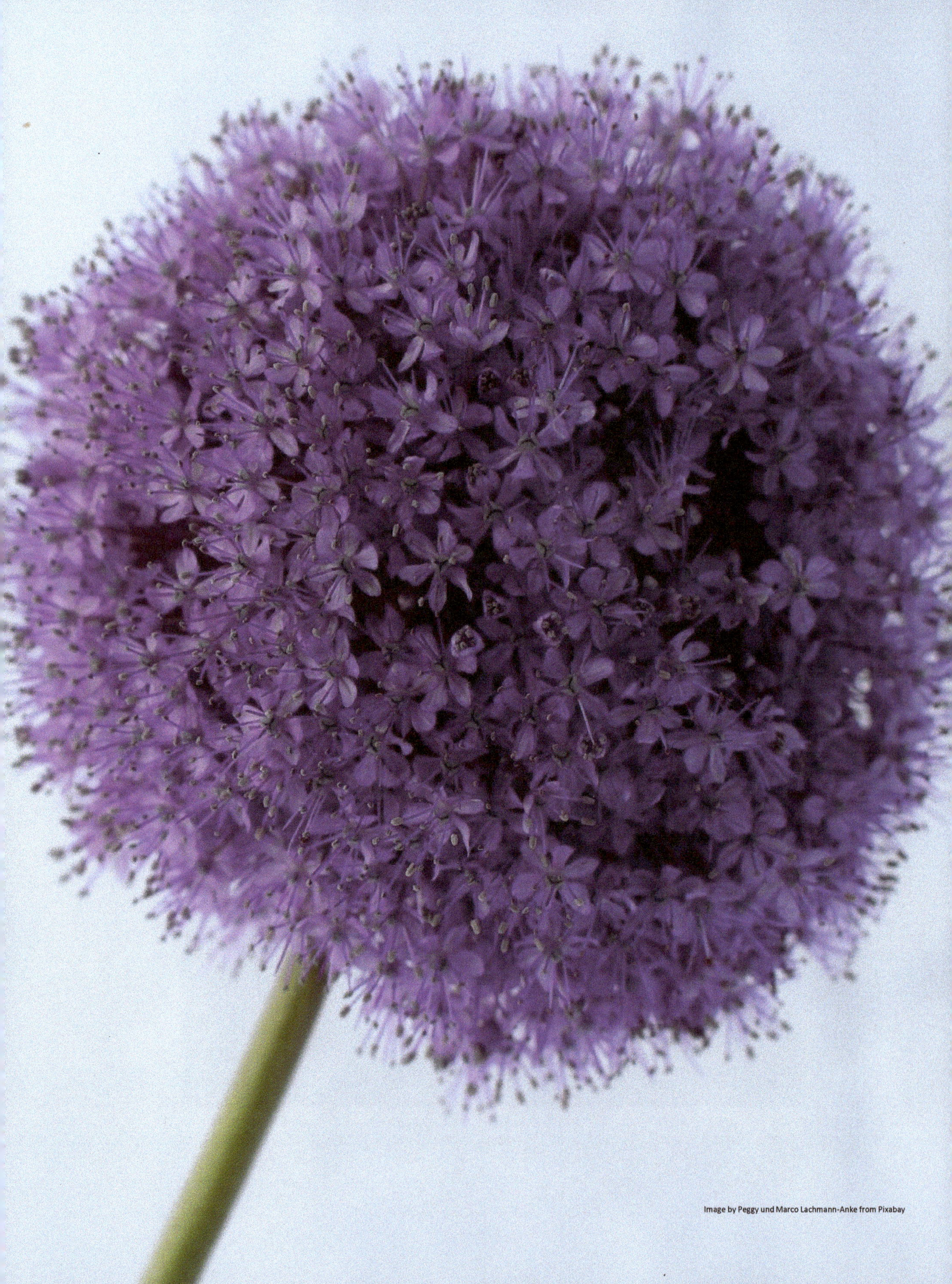

Image by Peggy und Marco Lachmann-Anke from Pixabay

Onion - Allium cepa

The humble onion Allium cepa has been used throughout history and became pan-global centuries ago. It is believed that the origin of the plant was in Iran, however this is difficult to know for certain due to its long history of use. The ancient Egyptians revered to the plant as it was used in embalming processes, and archaeological studies have shown that onions may have been common in China more than 5000 years ago. Relatives of onions are garlic, shallots, leeks, and chives. What is less known about the humble bulb is its long use as a natural medicine used for all manner of ailments and injuries by many ancient and contemporary cultures.

Onions are a rich source of sulphides and other compounds that are being studied. They are also rich in vitamins such as B1, B2, B6, vitamin C and vitamin E. As can be seen from the list of vitamins, it would be safe to assume that onion may be useful in the treatment of depression. However, the validated effectiveness of the extract made from the leaves and bulb is far greater than these simple vitamins would be able to achieve. Therefore, the other compounds found in the plant must also aid in the alleviation of depressive like symptoms. A brief list of some of the active sulfur compounds are alliin, allicin, ajoene, allyl propyl disulfide, diallyl trisulfide (DATS), S-allylcysteine (SAC), vinyldithiins and sallylmercaptocysteine. The presence of prostaglandins in onions is also interesting because these compounds are potent anti-inflammatory and vasodilators.

A great deal of research has been undertaken to understand the antidepressant actions of onions and in a paper released in 2016 it was shown that fresh juice of onion displayed significant anti-inflammatory actions as well as a reduction in acute and chronic pain. Research conducted in Japan in 2007 also had positive results in the management of depression by merely giving onion powder (50 mg per kilo of body weight) a day. This paper used the standard drug imipramine as a comparative treatment in the testing, and it was found that onion powder was as effective if not more effective that the use of imipramine. Research from 2009 showed that onion extract also influences the levels of testosterone in the body by measured increases, whilst at the same time had a positive effect on sperm motility and viability. This is good news if you're a man and depressed about not being able to start a family.

A side effect of being depressed and lethargic due to the pointlessness of it all, is the inevitable gain in weight of sufferers. The simple onion is proving useful as it has been shown that a diet high in onion inhibits the processing of lipids or fats. In various research papers, the outcome or results supported the claims that onions aid in the reduction of weight. As a result, the use of the humble onion in the diet of depression sufferers may also make you happier and skinnier at the same time.

Several clinical trials recommend a regime of high onion diet or daily juice to be continued for at least 14 days before assessing the effectiveness.

So, our provincial forebears in Europe, Asia and the middle east were probably far more content with their lots due to diets high in these miraculous plants. One such dish we can therefore recommend is the provincial classic onion soup. Not only will it improve your mood but also reduce weight, increase testosterone levels, and fight infections.

[1] S. M. Miri and A. Roughani, "Allium species growing in Iran: Chemical compositions and pharmacological activity Allium species growing in Iran : Chemical compositions and pharmacological activity," no. September, 2018.

[2] M. Marrelli, V. Amodeo, G. Statti, and F. Conforti, "Biological Properties and Bioactive Components of Allium cepa L .: Focus on Potential Benefits in the Treatment of Obesity and Related Comorbidities," 2019.

[3] R. K. Upadhyay, "Nutraceutical, pharmaceutical and therapeutic uses of," vol. 2016, no. 1, pp. 46–64, 2016.

[4] R. Mousavi, Z. H. Fashi, M. H. Jahromy, and R. Rasooli, "iMedPub Journals Potential of the Allium jesdianum Extract in Suppression of Anxiety and Depression in Mice Keywords:," pp. 1–5, 2017.

[5] N. Samad, F. Yasmin, M. A. Shahzad, M. M. Ayaz, and D. Saleem, "Nootropic and Anti-Stress Effects of Allium Cepa Bulb and Quercetin in Male Mice," pp. 1–7, 2019.

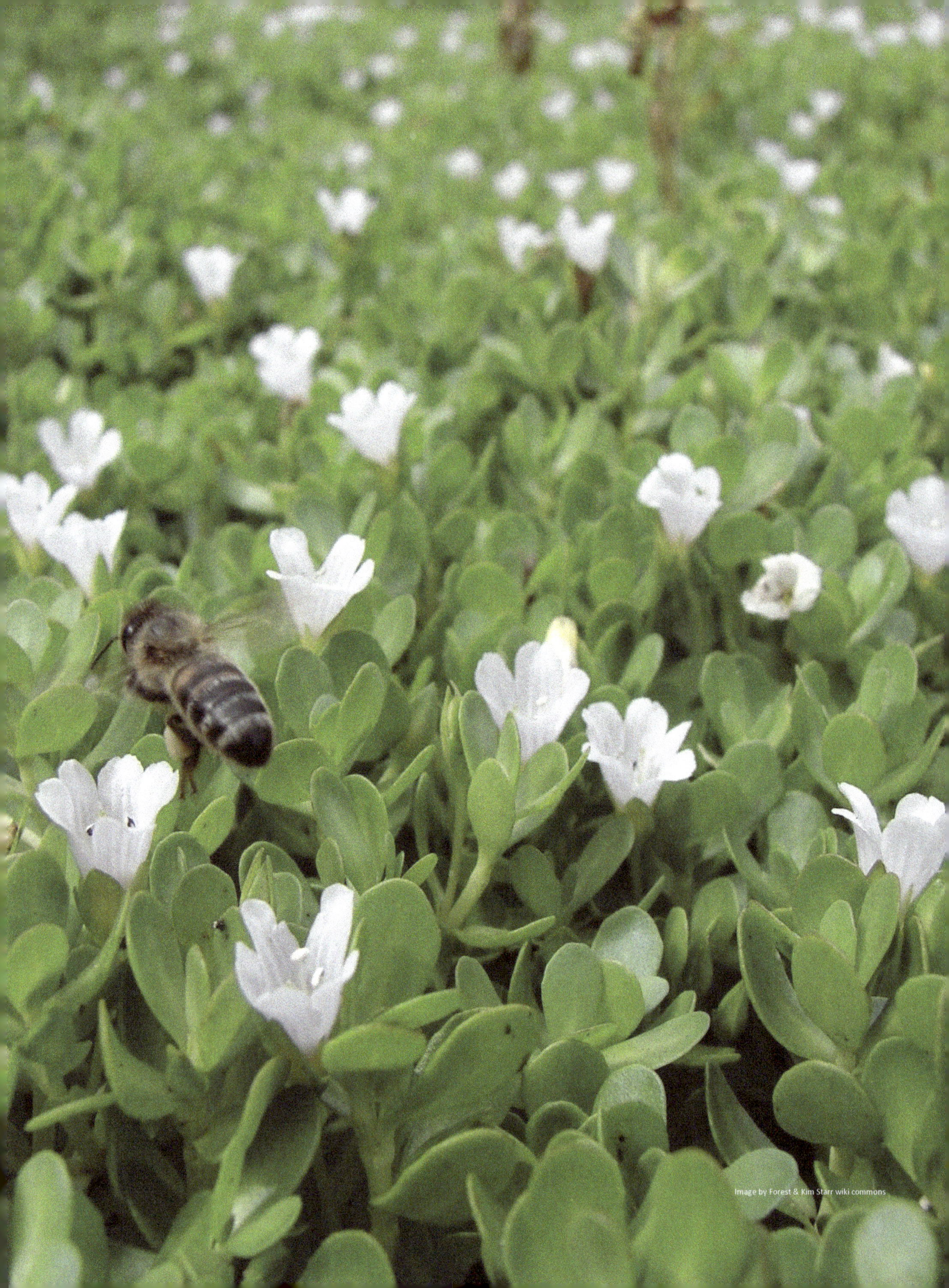

Image by Forest & Kim Starr wiki commons

Water hyssop - Bacopa monnieri

Bacopa monnieri is found throughout Asia and other tropical zones in the world such as those in Australia, Florida, Hawaii, South America, Africa, Madagascar, and the Caribbean. This plant is a genuinely pan-tropical citizen. Water hyssop, as its name implies, is a semi-aquatic plant preferring bogs, marshes and even surviving quite well on top of the water. There is some confusion in one of its local names Brahmi herb, as this is also shared with Gotu Kola (Centella asiatica).

Bacopa has been used in Ayurvedic medicine for thousands of years and is considered one of the main medicinal herbs in this system. Traditionally it is used as anxiety, epileptic disorders, dementia, blood purifier, cough and rheumatism, dermatitis, anaemia, diabetes, promote fertility, and prevent miscarriage. However, the traditional claim that the herb is useful in supporting the central nervous system and brain function is of most interest to us here.

In 2015, a trial was conducted to verify the antidepressant actions of the herb. In this trial, the researchers used a methanol/water extraction of the leaves from the plant and found that, at doses of 200 mg/kg body weight in the test animals, a significant improvement in the depression markers was seen. The effect was comparable to the standard drug imipramine.

A research article published in the "International Journal of Basic & Clinical Pharmacology" in 2016 also sought to understand the mechanism through which Bacopa monnieri had its antidepressant effect. In this article, the standard antidepressant drug fluoxetine was used as a comparative measure. The researchers found that the ethanol extract of the plant had similar effects as fluoxetine. They further tested the extract on the monoamine serotonin and its role in the aetiology of depression. It was found that the bacosides, unique compounds of bacopa, did influence levels of serotonin in the test animals. As a result, the ethanol extract was shown to influence serotonin levels and did not influence motor activity in the test animals, which indicates the plant is not a psychoactive drug.

It is interesting to note that the plant has long been used in traditional medicine for the treatment of memory loss and dementia. A more recent study in 2019 from Malaysia showed that the bacosides were significantly neuronal protective and actually prevented amyloid-beta build up in plaque material on the neurons in the brain, which is a symptom of Alzheimer's disease. This research also showed that Bacopa monnieri had anti-inflammatory and antioxidant properties which are both associated with the lessening of dementia and depression as inflammation of the central nervous system is a causative factor in both.

Additional studies, one from Italy and another from Australia, showed that a dose of 300 mg/kg per day significantly improved memory in all test subjects. A trial in Melbourne Victoria Australia showed that a higher single dose of the ethanol extract from the Water hyssop was shown to permanently increase cognitive ability in a test group aged between 18 – 44 years.

All in all, a very useful botanical for depression and brain function.

[1] M. A. Mannan, A. B. Abir, and M. R. Rahman, "Antidepressant-like effects of methanolic extract of Bacopa monnieri in mice," BMC Complement. Altern. Med., vol. 15, no. 1, 2015.

[2] C. Girish, S. Oommen, and R. Vishnu, "Evidence for the involvement of the monoaminergic system in the antidepressant-like activity of methanolic extract of Bacopa monnieri in albino mice," Int. J. Basic Clin. Pharmacol., vol. 5, no. 3, pp. 914–922, 2016.

[3] A. S. Abdul Manap et al., "Bacopa monnieri, a Neuroprotective Lead in Alzheimer Disease: A Review on Its Properties, Mechanisms of Action, and Preclinical and Clinical Studies," Drug Target Insights, vol. 13, 2019.

Virtual depression

"The difference between technology and slavery is that slaves are fully aware that they are not free"

Nassim Nicholas Taleb

On Thursday the 12th of November 2020 Google search engine took a little more than half a second to show over 296 million hits to the question "Does the internet cause depression?" The answer appears to be ... yes!

It is surprising that researchers have been looking at psychological impacts of internet use shortly after the internet was transformed into the worldwide web. It is believed that the internet became open to the general public in or around 1989 and that the first clinic specialising in internet addiction (IA) was set up just over five years later in 1995. And only three years later, the IA scale was developed in 1998 by Dr Kimberly Young at the Bonaventure university in New York. At first, it was mainly computer games and programming that occupied internet addicts. Today, addiction is largely associated with social media platforms. These platforms appear to have an effect on the psychology and physiology of addicts in much the same way as heroin or alcohol addiction. And yes, a Social Media Addiction Scale was developed in 2015. There is even a Cyber Loafing Scale (CLS) that is used to assess employees who waste time surfing the internet and not doing what they are paid for. With the release of the first Apple iPhone in 2007 things became worse as it allowed users to surf the web on a handheld device in a seamless manner like never before. A large study conducted in South Korea in 2018 resulted in a new category of IA aptly named 'smartphone addiction'. It was far worse than the plain vanilla addiction of personal computers and laptops. One reason for the severity of smartphone addiction is relatively easy to understand because these appliances remain turned on and accompany us twenty-four hours a day, enabling the owner to have constant access to the web. In 2007, IA was defined as a person spending between 8.5 and up to 21 hours per week actively on a screen. This criterion is no longer relevant to smartphone use as they are now with us day and night making it virtually impossible to predict the total amount of time spent on them. In 2018 Apple introduced Screen Time app as a parental control feature. Researchers have tried to answer this question of IA and have established a figure of approximately three and a half hours per day is spent on mobile phones by the average user. So, an average mobile phone user spends over 24 hours in a week, or a day and night continually in front of a screen.

This topic is not a revelation to most people. Yet, people under the age of thirty might find it a revelation that they have a 50% chance of being addicted or almost one in two people are potentially smartphone addicts. There has been the invention of a clinical term known as 'nomophobia' which literally means fear of not having a smartphone. Related to this is the fear of missing out known as 'FOMO'.

In other forms of addiction, we often hear "I'm not addicted, I know how to control it", or "I can stop anytime I want to." When hearing these types of statements, we could think of denial, and that the user is already addicted. In 2014, a meta-analysis of research into IA from thirty-one nations it was found that the overall prevalence of IA was around 6%. Needless to say, this number is concerning, to say the least as it indicates that as many as four hundred million people are addicted to the internet if we were to extrapolate this into the global population - and keeping in mind that only 51% of the world's population has access to the internet. This is three times the prevalence of compulsive gambling which is estimated to be less than 2%. It gets worse when we consider that the internet only really came into being in the mid-1990s. So, a young adult prior to this time was not influenced as much as the Millennial Generation who commenced their reign in 1994. Findings in regions such as China, South Korea, India and Japan, IA is estimated to be as high as 40% in that generation alone. I am sure you can begin to see a possible correlation between Smartphone Addiction and the meteoric increase in depression throughout our societies.

To make matters more complicated, the internet became much more deadly (a word chosen with care as more suicides are being attributed to Social Media Syndrome) due to the arrival of Facebook in 2004. Prior, AI was primarily a hobby of gamers, but with the arrival of social media the peace was disturbed and reality was rapidly discarded for fantasy as online marketers, silicone influencers, trolls and cyberbullies were just some of the new organisms evolving into this strange new world.

Prior to Facebook and its brethren, IA tended to be the realm of introverts and intellectual nerds who, after spending far too much time playing games or programming random sequences of code, found themselves isolated and even more alone which had the result of causing depression. It was simply too much time spent on solo pursuits. However, a terrifying aspect of the emerging new world order is its ability to tell you how ineffectual and ugly you are as people now compare themselves to faceless others. Perhaps not in so many words, but as we follow handsome jet setting studs, the inference is that we follow them because we wish to be like them. We follow the family of shallow petty reality stars because they seem more real than our empty lives. We follow the political advice from the online magazine or paper that we have always read. We follow relationship advice from a person on the other side of the world who may have been divorced twice. We follow recipes. We follow fashion. We follow health advice..........in short 'we follow!'.

Studies have shown that even those people who appear to be the most successful and happiest on social media are in fact some of the most at-risk people due to the adoption of personas that are false, and the constant work required to maintain them and the fantasy. We can all now have meaningless casual sex by swiping right or left. We can purchase nearly anything immediately and end up with our lives filled with rubbish that has not made a micron shift in our happiness. Or conversely, if we are poor, we are able to see the lives of the rich and vacuous and everything that we are missing out on. Then we turn to religion online to save our souls only to find yet another empty charade of power-hungry new age preachers.

David Bowie, in a BBC interview in 1999, stated "The potential of what the internet is going to do to society, both good and bad, is unimaginable. We're on the cusp of something both exhilarating and terrifying!" He was not sure in exactly in what manner this would evolve, and I am sure that today we can see the terrifying aspect of the internet and social media that he spoke of. What was once designed to connect people, and free them from ignorance is now disconnecting people and overwhelming them with the ignorance of wrong information. However, when a person is depressed, alone and insecure, the internet is quite possibly irresistible. It may be the only form of relationship people have. Teaching them that life is full of shallow relationships, quick click gratification, and, that once eyes stray from the screen and gaze at the reality around us, to only find that it has become so dull and boring in comparison to the magical world of a digital lobotomy.

Aligned with the overuse of laptops and smartphones is the emerging threat of electromagnetic damage users are now suffering from. Naturally, internet service providers, social media content providers and advertising companies will endeavour to discredit any discussion on this topic with a wave of a hand and saying, 'all unsubstantiated rubbish!'. Paper after paper is drawing links between handheld electronic devices and depression. As far back as 2011, the World Health Organisation published scientific work on radio frequency, alluding to a possible link to glioma tumours which are a common form of brain cancer. Other research studies explore links associating handheld phones, with causing headaches, lethargy, memory loss, and disturbed sleep patterns.

All in all, the excessive use of smartphones is gaining a very negative reputation. However, the word 'excessive' is all we need to consider. The internet and smartphones have changed our societies in a short period of time. The benefits are many, and the impacts on how we go about our lives, for the most part, is positive. It is the overuse of the technology that leads to a multitude of health and emotional issues. As with all things, in moderation technology is astounding. But what is moderation when our work, social and family lives have become saturated with the click and swipe?

Most of our communication today is more meaningless and more massive. A simple email or post can produce numerous replies, responses and comments, all of which expect us to respond to—an endless loop of communication. We can end up in a constant stream of meaningless responses, hits click-throughs. when a simple reply to a question is all that is needed. Needless to say, this vacuum of activity flows in our private and work lives. Do they bring meaning, enrich our lives to make our it special in the long run?

We now look for validation of our lives from strangers on social media platforms, from 'likes' on Facebook to professional endorsements on LinkedIn, our intrinsic understanding of our value is being controlled by faceless people and not by our close peers and friends.

In a survey carried out by a company known as Surecall in America, over one thousand people were asked a set of questions. The findings were both surprising and worrying. Of those people interviewed 10% admitted to checking their phones during sex. Also, the people who slept with their phones beside their beds 30% admitted to fear and anxiety if they did not have their phone. 17% admitted that they were dissatisfied with their lives, and 21% admitted to feelings of general sadness. As a result, the simple act of placing your phone in another room while you sleep will have a beneficial impact on your life.

There are other tricks, or 'hacks' researchers have found to reduce our dependence on our smartphones. These are:

Delete all unnecessary Apps on your phone.

Restrict when you check your social media status to possible on two or three times per day. Your friends can wait. If they can't, then they are not friends, and you are better off without them.

Buy an alarm clock instead of using your phone close to your bed.

Turn the phone to greyscale. It will work just as good, but it will not be as visually appealing.

Make at least some time, every day, phone free. Don't take your phone to the gym or when you go for a walk. If you need music, then get another music device.

Stop taking photos of everything. If you think about all the images on your phone, most of them are never looked at again after the first time.

Turn off notifications. If you know of Pavlov's dog, then you will understand why. If you don't know then look him up.

But most of all, in your downtime interact with real people, your family and friends. However, if you find them lacking because you either don't have many or you are geographically distant from them, then join a club or society.

If all else is simply too difficult then take your dog or by now any form of mascot out of your door to the nearest café with magazines, fresh juices and a warm pavement or windowsill for your friend to sleep on.

[1] Y. J. Kim, H. M. Jang, Y. Lee, D. Lee, and D. J. Kim, 'Effects of internet and Smartphone addictions on depression and anxiety based on propensity score matching analysis,' Int. J. Environ. Res. Public Health, vol. 15, no. 5, pp. 1–10, 2018.

[2] C. Cheng and A. Y. L. Li, 'Internet addiction prevalence and quality of (real) life: A meta-Analysis of 31 nations across seven world regions,' Cyberpsychology, Behav. Soc. Netw., vol. 17, no. 12, pp. 755–760, 2014.

[3] S. Ahmad Bhat and M. Hussain Kawa, 'A Study of Internet Addiction and Depression among University Students,' Int. J. Behav. Res. Psychol., no. October, pp. 105–108, 2015.

[4] M. Koç, 'Internet addiction and psychopatology,' Turkish Online J. Educ. Technol., vol. 10, no. 1, pp. 143–148, 2011.

[5] İ. TAŞ, 'Association between depression, anxiety, stress, social support, resilience and internet addiction: a structural equation modelling,' Malaysian Online J. Educ. Technol., vol. 7, no. 3, pp. 1–10, 2019.

[6] A. Akin and M. İskender, 'Internet Addiction and Depression, Anxiety and Stress,' Int. Online J. Educ. Sci., vol. 3, no. 1, pp. 138–148, 2011.

[7] P. Effects et al., 'Problematic smartphone use - Wikipedia.'.

[8] S. A. Bahrainian, K. Haji Alizadeh, M. R. Raeisoon, O. Hashemi Gorji, and A. Khazaee, 'Relationship of Internet addiction with self-esteem and depression in university students,' J. Prev. Med. Hyg., vol. 55, no. 3, pp. 86–89, 2014.

[9] T. Ayas and M. B. Horzum, 'Relation Between Depression, Loneliness, Self-Esteem and Internet Addiction,' Education, vol. 133, no. 3, pp. 283–291, 2007.

[10] D. Kim, Y. Lee, J. Lee, J. E. K. Nam, and Y. Chung, 'Development of Korean Smartphone Addiction Proneness Scale for youth,' PLoS One, vol. 9, no. 5, pp. 1–8, 2014.

[11] C. Şahın, 'The predictive level of social media addiction for life satisfaction: A study on university students,' Turkish Online J. Educ. Technol., vol. 2017, no. December Special IssueINTE, pp. 515–520, 2017.

[12] R. L. Blasco, C. L. Cosculluela, and A. Q. Robres, 'Social network addiction and its impact on anxiety level among university students,' Sustain., vol. 12, no. 13, 2020.

[13] M. Kwon, D. J. Kim, H. Cho, and S. Yang, 'The smartphone addiction scale: Development and validation of a short version for adolescents,' PLoS One, vol. 8, no. 12, 2013. [14] '6166494.'.

[15] SureCall, 'Cellphone Use In America,' p. 4, 2018.

[16] O. Orsal, O. Orsal, A. Unsal, and S. S. Ozalp, 'Evaluation of Internet Addiction and Depression among University Students,' Procedia - Soc. Behav. Sci., vol. 82, pp. 445–454, 2013.

[17] E. Dalbudak, C. Evren, S. Aldemir, K. S. Coskun, H. Ugurlu, and F. G. Yildirim, 'Relationship of internet addiction severity with depression, anxiety, and alexithymia, temperament and character in university students,' Cyberpsychology, Behav. Soc. Netw., vol. 16, no. 4, pp. 272–278, 2013.

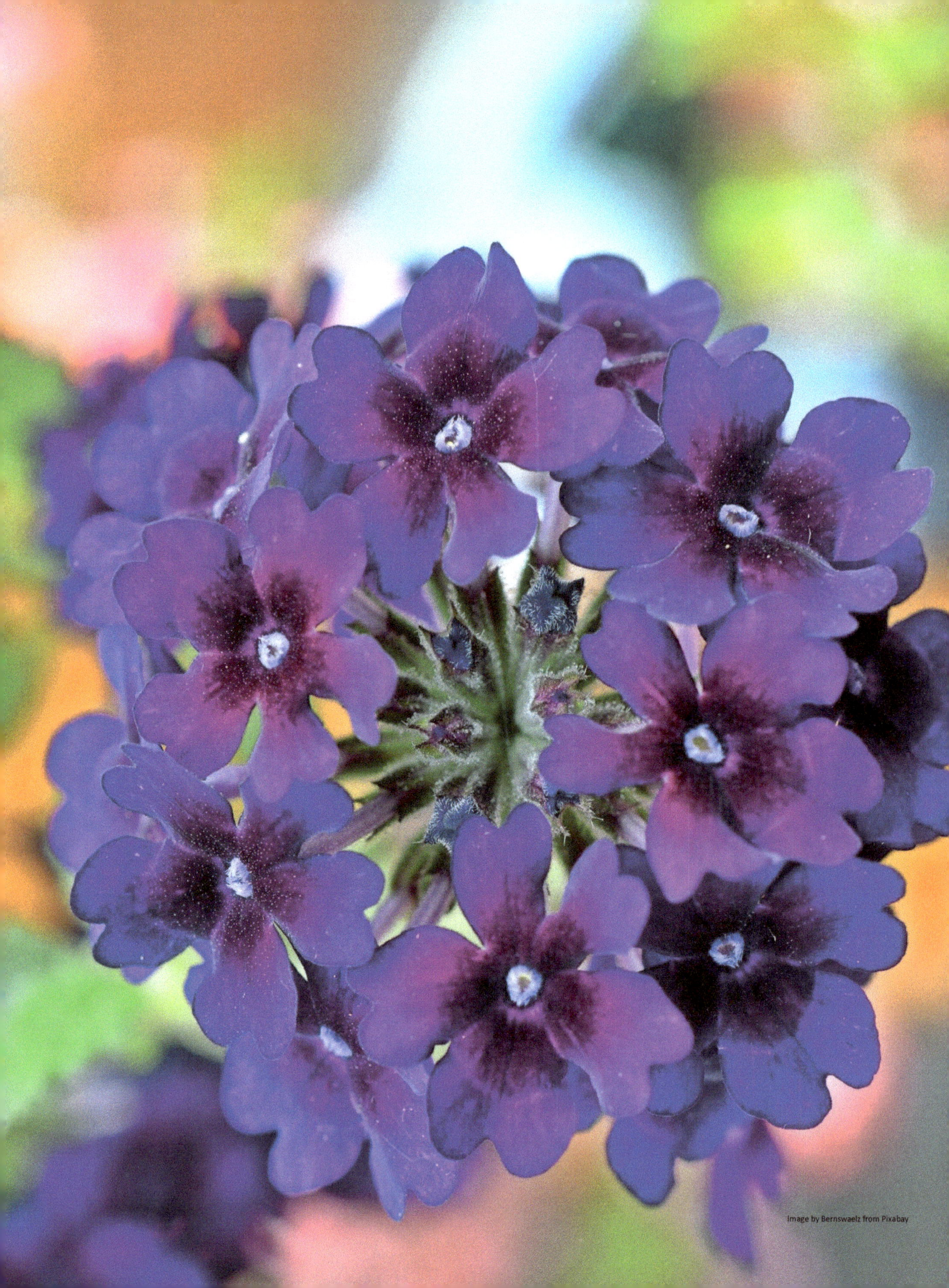

Image by Bernswaelz from Pixabay

Vervain - Verbena officinalis

Native to Europe this common weed has been used for a millennium, and all manner of spiritual and medicinal properties have been associated with this plant. It has commanded and possessed an important place in the ancient Greek and Roman empires. In Greek mythology, the herb was associated with the Titan Goddess Eos Erigenia, the goddess of the dawn, who rose every morning from her home at the edge of the ocean. The herb was known as 'Juno's tears' in Greece, and in Egypt it is known as 'Isis tears'. As we can see, the plant has been employed by all cultures throughout Europe and into North Africa. In Christian mythology, the wounds Christ suffered during his crucifixion were staunched by Verbena. It therefore has long been associated with warding off evil spirits, and in the middle ages for warding off witches. Ironically, it is also used in occult preparations such as the Mandragora spell.

In modern times it is still a prevalent medicinal herb. It is highly popular in Europe as it is included in the many texts on herbal medicine ranging from Culpeper's Herbal (1652) to today's books on herbal medicine. Verbena Officinalis is now found across the globe.

Clinical research into the antidepressant actions of the herb was carried out in 2015 in India. It was found in the trial that a dose of 300 mg/kg body weight had comparable antidepressant results to the standard drug imipramine. A 2016 study from Pakistan tested as to whether the herb was effective in the treatment of anxiety, insomnia and convulsions. It was found that the herb promoted sleep and reduced convulsions. As the herb possesses sedative-like actions, the anxiety aspect of the study also had a positive outcome. The standard drug used during this trial was diazepam, which was only slightly better than Verbena leaf extract at doses of 300 mg/kg body weight. Another study, this time from Serbia in 2017, found that Verbena officinalis had similar results when compared to paroxetine as the comparative antidepressant drug.

There are many clinical trials on the effectiveness of Verbena in the management of mild to moderate depression. However, the herb is also a sedative, so care should be taken when using it.

The active compounds unique to the plant are verbenalin and verbascoside. Other compounds found in the plant are sculletelarein, apigenin, luteolin, quercetin, and kaempferol. However, as is common in the study of botanical medicines and their actions, at present it is still unclear exactly how the extract from the plant interacts with the human body to achieve the positive results. It is assumed that the ethanolic extract of the plant influences the serotonin, dopamine and norepinephrine modulation.

In the past and across cultures, it has many historical references to its use as an oracle stimulant to promote vivid dreams and represent omens for the future.

[1] T. Jawaid, S. A. Imam, and M. Kamal, "Antidepressant activity of methanolic extract of Verbena Officinalis Linn. plant in mice," Asian J. Pharm. Clin. Res., vol. 8, no. 4, pp. 308–310, 2015.

[2] A. W. Khan, A. U. Khan, and T. Ahmed, "Anticonvulsant, anxiolytic, and sedative activities of Verbena officinalis," Front. Pharmacol., vol. 7, no. DEC, pp. 1–8, 2016.

[3] 江小, "No Title网空间服务业: 效率、约束及发展前景* ———以体育和文化产业为例," 經濟研究, vol. 2, no. 5, pp. 208–209, 2018.

[4] S. C. Hood, "Verbena officinalis," Pharm. Biol., vol. 15, no. 4, p. 212, 1977.

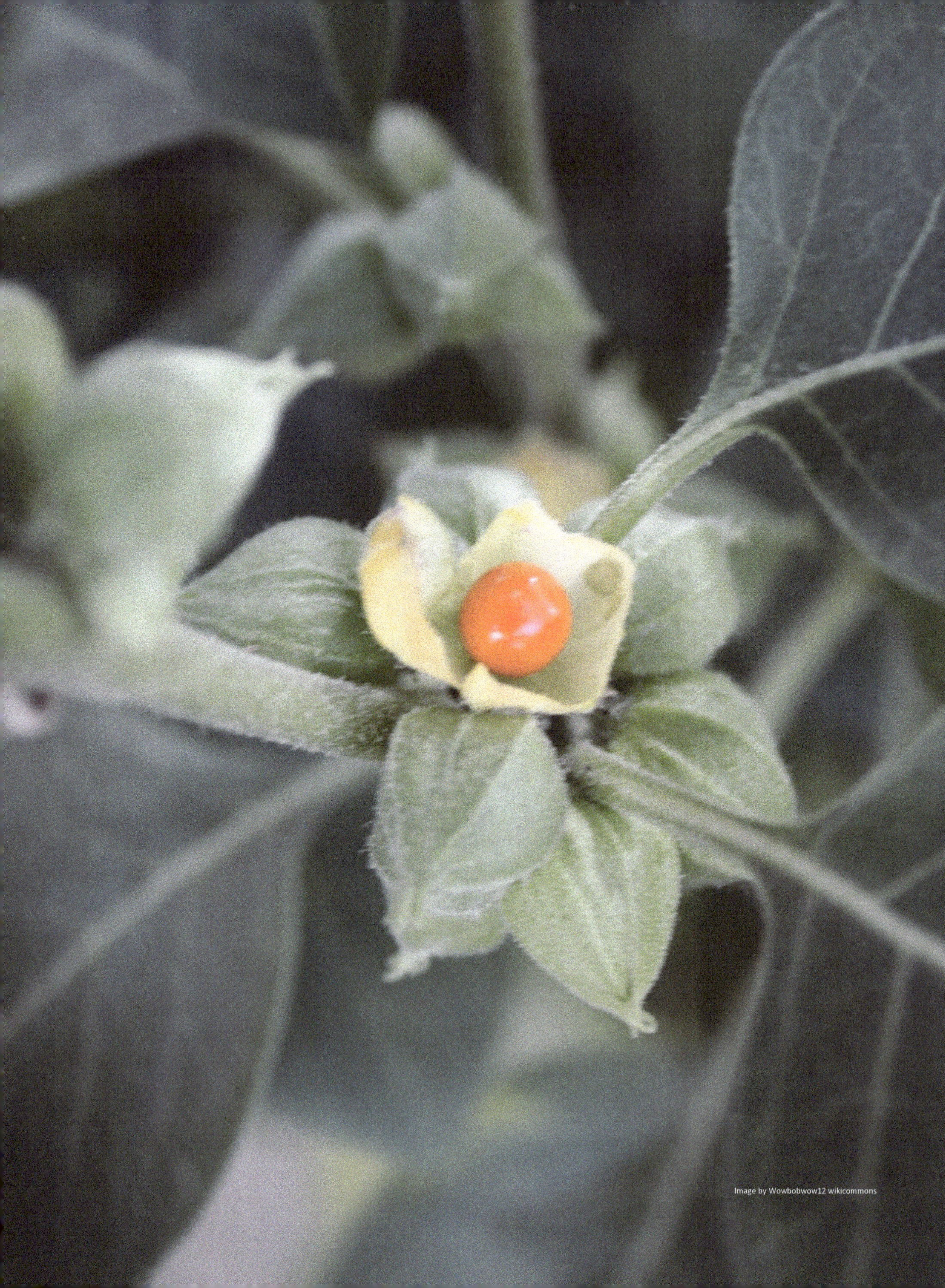

Image by Wowbobwow12 wikicommons

Ashwagandha - Withania somnifera

Withania somnifera has for thousands of years been used in both Unani and Ayurvedic systems of medicine. Some reports state that it has been used for at least 3,000 years. It is considered to be one of the main herbs in these systems for its life extension properties. In so saying, Ashwagandha is considered to be an 'adaptogen' herb, which roughly translated means "A medicine that aids in the ability to endure stress". As a result, we could easily state that all the herbs contained within this book are also adaptogens. The plant has been studied extensively with the main chemical compounds unique to Ashwagandha labelled as "withanolides", and it was found it had similar properties to the compounds found in Ginseng, and thereby resulting in the other name for the plant, Indian Ginseng.

It is found in the Northern regions of India and across the Arabian region to Yemen on the Arabian Peninsula.

The roots are the main part of the plant used in traditional medicine. Claims that it is an anti-inflammatory, nootropic (brain function improvement), antibacterial, anti-ulcer and general tonic have all been supported in clinical studies. The most interesting use of the plant is in the treatment of senile dementia and bronchial asthma equally, which may be due to the anti-inflammatory actions of the herb in both brain tissue and epithelial regions of the bronchia.

When reviewing the research carried out on its anti-anxiety and antidepressant actions, we find various reports all substantiating these claims. One report from a clinical trial carried out in Iran in 2014 showed that doses of 400 mg/kg body weight of the water extract of the roots significantly reduced the nitric acid levels in the brain tissue of test mice. Nitric acid is a gaseous signaling compound found in the mammalian brain, and elevated levels of nitric acid is associated with stress and anxiety. Therefore, a reduction in nitric acid and ensuing inflammatory response in the brain tissue of test subjects is evidence of the effectiveness of the herb in reducing depression and anxiety. In a trial, the root extract was compared to fluoxetine, a standard anti-depression drug, and concluded that the extract did lessen the symptoms of stress and depression significantly, but it was not as effective as fluoxetine.

There was a burst of research into the use of Ashwagandha as a depression moderating medicine in the period 1999-2001 with all papers supporting the use. In this period, the standard synthetic drugs used as comparative measures were mainly imipramine and lorazepam. A more recent clinical trial in 2015 sought to compare the root extract to the standard drug imipramine and found whilst the root extract was once again highly effective in the reduction of depression and anxiety it was marginally less effective than imipramine.

Whilst the synthetic drugs outperformed Withania somnifera, the plant had a raft of additional health benefits which makes it more advantageous. These are cardiac tonic, anticancer, anti-inflammatory, memory and cognitive function, antibacterial, and analgesic. Also, there are few side effects with the Ashwagandha, and it is considered to be nontoxic.

[1] P. Bharathi, V. Seshayamma, G. H. Jagannadharao, and N. Sivakumar, "Evaluation of Antidepressant Activity of Aqueous Extract of Withania Somnifera [Aswagandha] Roots in Albino Mice," IOSR J. Pharm. Biol. Sci. Ver, vol. 10, no. 1, pp. 2319–7676, 2015.

[2] M. Attari, F. Jamaloo, S. Shadvar, N. Fakhraei, and A. R. Dehpour, "Effect of withania somnifera dunal root extract on behavioral despair model in mice: A possible role for nitric oxide," Acta Med. Iran., vol. 54, no. 3, pp. 165–172, 2016.

[3] A. Constituents, "Monograph. Withania somnifera.," Altern. Med. Rev., vol. 9, no. 2, pp. 211–214, 2004.

Training your black dog

"Knowledge requires effort. Wisdom requires pain"

Paul Evers

Thanks to Sir Winston Churchill we have a black dog as mascot to keep us company in our dungeons of emptiness. However, Winston chose and equally dark and depressing friend for his walks of gloom. This does not mean we have to follow in his weary footsteps. We can choose whatever manifestation our mascots should be. What animal best suits us. It is quite understandable that a dark colour in the beginning may be more in tune with how we feel, yet over time this hopefully changes, and our mascots can take on more vivid and uplifting hues. Therefore, you have the opportunity to transform or personalise your mascot into any animal you fancy. From a chihuahua to a wolf, or perhaps a black sarcastic duck is more your flavour. Whatever you choose, it may be highly beneficial to have an external focal point for your depression and imbue this mascot with its own personality, tastes or colour. As a result, it may destabilise your current situation just enough for you to make positive changes for your future. Whimsical as this may be, this will be extremely useful as you combine all the discussed facets that connect to your black dog so that you develop your own unique coping mechanisms.

We discussed facets backed by research that a depressive person withdraws and will isolate themselves regardless of how many people are physically around them. If a depressed person can create such private world, then it should not be too hard to create an imaginary friend. In this creative process we begin to reverse the disconnection process via projecting our silent internal dialogues onto an external focal point with our mascot.

The longer a person suffers from depression the more they reduce their footprint on the world as if they are folding into themselves. A diminishing origami of the soul. So, in order to get control of your depression you will need to begin to unfold and open up what was previously hidden and protected. Risk must be liberally sprinkled on your breakfast cereal. What was previously severed and disconnected slowly over time must now be reconnected with. This is not a fast process in fact it should be a very slow process.

It is this reaching out and reconnecting to segments of our lives that we have diminished or made to disappear, will connect you back with friends, sports, music, family, education, hobbies, eating and maybe even sex with someone else. Yet the important piece of advice is to not enter into a manic period and make yourself reconnect with everything all at once as this will surely create confusion and exhaustion. Rather choose one segment and take your time.

Depression is unavoidable if you have the tendency. We cannot say, "Not now, I'm busy come back tomorrow." All that can be done is to recognise the oncoming wave of grey weight and wait for it to arrive in its full force. However, we can decide how we interact with this wave. The clear message that has come out of the vast amounts of research into this ever-growing medical condition globally, is that one therapy or drug is insufficient to address all the contributing factors that result in creating depressive episodes or how long they may last. Antidepressants prescribed by our doctors and therapists are undeniably useful, yet they may bring on undesirable side effects or are not effective for everyone. Art therapy may work for you and then not for her. To be able to have control and be able to tailor a daily regime, unique to you, will however be invaluable.

The acquisition of knowledge is in itself the acquisition of control, and in this case the power to influence your depression. A sufferer who has no idea how or why they suffer from depression is akin to a child set adrift in a small boat on a vast ocean, and in effect powerless. Yet if that child knew of tides and currents, how to make a sail or any number of skills that will allow it to manipulate the boat, then that knowledge or skill set is of enormous impact. It is the same with our depressions. Our diet, or lack of it, the chosen music, and the colours we surround ourselves with, will all have either a positive or negative impact on how we navigate the vast oceans of ennui that make up the world of the depressed, and the non-depressed.

The primary task is to accept that our black dogs will not disappear merely if we tell them to. Our mascots are going to be around us for weeks, months and even years. The best strategy is to get to know this new external mascot. Apply personality to it, even give it a name, a colour, favourite music, hobby, sound and learn when it wants to play or simply sit and stare at you. Struggling against depression in most cases makes it worse because our we are our opponent. We fight against our image in a mirror, knowing exactly every move, every thought of our reflection. So, make your depression work for you. Use your mascot wisely. Address the positives coming through instead of the negatives.

There is one golden rule that must be used at all times. Whatever you choose whatever you do, and whatever herb you utilise, once commenced I recommend they must be maintained for a minimum of 14 days before you can discard one for another. As we have discussed, it takes about this long for therapy to show effectiveness. So, if you are using for instance *Melissa officinalis* as a tisane then continue drinking it for two weeks before changing to a Rosemary tisane. Secondly, do keep notes, lots and lots of notes, because these will help refine your approach to living with your black dog.

A critical thing we have to do is accept things the way they are. It is this decision, to accept it as the bedrock of your new world. As the American author and commentator, Steve Maraboli, has said "Acceptance makes an incredibly fertile soil for the seeds of change". Therefore, accept that you are depressed and that you are not the only one. Many of the people around may also be suffering from depression and like you, they feel that they must hide it. As a result, your claims that no one understands you may be how a person close to you thinks about you. That you do not understand them and vice versa. Accept your depression, and do not be afraid to discuss it openly. And accept that you are probably far more intelligent than you give yourself credit for. Accept that you can change the status quo for the better.

Enjoy training and walking your unique mascot. Personalize it with a voice, and scent, give it a hobby, feed it well, dress it differently, paint its house, step onto the grass, forget meaningless communication and most of all have loud intense arguments with it.

Herbs

The herbs in this book can permeate all aspects of your daily life, from consuming a simple tisane/tea to its use as an essential oil in perfume. The table below outlines the herbs and how to use them. How you can manufacture your own is discussed in the next chapter.

Caution however not to use too many herbs at one time as this will create confusion as to which one works for you and which does not. Therefore, integrate only one or a maximum of two at a time, and employ them consistently for no less than two weeks before changing to another herb.

The table informs that for instance *Melissa officinalis* can be used as an extract, tisane, essential aromatic oil and as a food. Others are best taken merely as an extract, as is the case with *Passiflora incarnata,* or *Aquilaria crassna* is best to be taken as an aromatic oil.

Herb	**Extract**	**Tisane**	**Oil**	**Food**
Abies pindrow	✓			
Allium jesdianum	✓			✓
Apium Graveolens	✓	✓		✓
Aquilaria crassna			✓	
Bacopa monnieri	✓			
Bupleurum falcatum	✓			
Centella asiatica	✓	✓		✓
Chrysopogon zizanioides	✓			
Citrus limon	✓	✓	✓	✓
Clitoria ternatea	✓	✓		
Coriandrum sativum	✓			✓
Crocus sativa	✓			✓
Cuminum cynimum	✓			✓
Curcumin longa	✓			✓
Dacus carota	✓			
Eichhornia crassipes	✓			
Ficus	✓			✓
Gastrodia elata	✓			
Griffonia simplicifolia	✓			
Hemerocallis citrina	✓	✓		
Hypericum perforatum	✓	✓		
Jasminum sambac	✓	✓	✓	
Magnolia	✓	✓	✓	
Melissa officinalis	✓	✓	✓	✓
Nordostachys jatamansi	✓		✓	
Ocimum sanctum	✓			✓
Paeonia	✓	✓		
Passiflora incarnata	✓			
Piper methysticum	✓	✓		
Rhodolia rosea	✓			
Rosmarinus officinalis	✓	✓	✓	✓
Tagetes erecta	✓		✓	
Valeriana officinalis	✓	✓		
Verbena officinalis	✓	✓	✓	
Viola odorata	✓	✓	✓	
Withania somnifera	✓			

Music
Review your musical choices. Stop listening to songs of unrequited love as they will feed your loneliness. Slash and Grunge music may give you an outlet for your anger, however, it will not resolve why you are angry in the first place. Background music will penetrate into your subconscious mind and reinforce the message that the artist is singing about. Rather choose uplifting instrumental music or music that empowers you.

Diet
Perhaps you have heard this quote before, regardless, it is still worth using when we discuss diet. According to urban myth, the native American Indians had this piece of wisdom; "Inside each of us are two wolves. One is darkness and despair, the other is light and hope. Which one will win? The answer of course is, the one you feed the most." This parable condenses the topic of diet. Begin with simple steps. Don't rush out and waste money purchasing the entire health food section of your local supermarket. All those groceries will most likely sit there and slowly spoil as you revert back to the instant gratification that junk food is so good at. Do purchase vitamins and minerals to bring about change. Give your body the necessary building blocks to commence the gradual improvement in overall health and mind. As you begin to take an interest in food as a medicine, you will be better able to incorporate foods in a well thought out and smooth process.

Colours
The discussion has clarified previously that colours play a subtle yet significant role in how we perceive the world. If you have surrounded yourself in dark and monotone decor, clothes and art, a variety of research has confirmed that this will work against you. Let's not suggest you should go wild with yellows and pinks, but choose more natural colours such as lighter blues, browns and greens. Stop wearing blacks, greys, dark colours. If your eyes are the windows to the soul, then let the soul look out from them onto refreshing views.

Hidden pollution
Take time to clean out the clutter of electronic devices and power supplies. Sitting in front of a computer screen or TV for hours on end will only make matters worse. Having bedside lights, an electric alarm clock, a television next to the bed will all have subtle impacts on your body. Your smartphone should be used to communicate in short concise conversations rather than holding the device close to your ear, and consequently your brain, for extended periods of time. Move from voice to text as much as possible. Get out into nature, no matter whether it is a small park close to your home or travelling to the countryside for a weekend detox. Try walking with bare feet and smell the unique aroma of nature as much as possible. Reconnect with your earth.

Exercise
Along with diet, exercise may be the best therapy you could engage in. Study after study has shown the powerful effect it has on the mind and spirit. You need to start in small steps remembering this is a consistent journey and not a mad race. Make simple easily attainable goals, such as the WTF technique; promise yourself before you go to bed that in the morning you will at least get changed into your exercise gear and stand outside your door, and to possibly have to say WTF I should go for a short walk at least. Another piece of wisdom is posed as a question "What is the difference between an expert and a novice?" The answer is "An expert has failed more times the novice has tried." Don't let self-image challenges stop you, because this will resolve as you repeat it again and again and again. In short, don't listen to all the excuses you have hidden away in your mind. Remember the man who stood in front of the firing squad "Just Do It!".

The internet

Every time you log onto the internet you are just like Alice disappearing down the rabbit hole into an unreal world. The mistake people make is thinking they can trust what they find on the internet, and this is in most cases completely untrue, especially when you try to judge yourself via the responses or advice from complete strangers. As Shakespeare wrote in King Lear "That way madness lies." Limit yourself to looking at your social media accounts to not more than three times per day or even less. By posting something once a day you will find that your friends and associates will know you are still alive, and a better quality of communication will follow. No one really wants to know what you ate for lunch or how upset you are that your favourite sitcom is no longer running. Worse, if they do care then they have emptier lives than you. Take up art, go to the gym or even better go for a walk in a forest, if you can without a cell network at all. Of all the recommendations this is the only one arguing for further disconnection rather than deeper connection. Disconnect from the internet and reconnect with the real world.

Friends

This segment can be quite tricky as you may not have any or the ones you have may not be good for you. Even family members may not be the best choice. Possibly the first friend you may come to depend on will be the one you have created as your mascot. An anti-friend so to speak. Reconnection with the outside world may just require the projection of part of your mind into it. New friends may be found through reconnecting with the world around you through exercise, hobbies or hiking in a forest. Do try not to establish the same type of friendships that you are actually wishing to leave behind as they were part of your depression. Discover you, be clear about who you are. If you manifest into what you think other people want, then they will not be able to relate or help you. Don't smile for the sake of smiling, as in time people will recognise the lie and label you as fake or plastic and avoid you. Simply remain you and rather be proud or your depression. Commence a conversation like "Hi I'm Charlie, I come here often as it helps with my depression and I really like cupcakes!". If the person runs away from you consider yourself immensely lucky. If they smile and say "I know what you mean!" it's probable that a far more beneficial friendship will grow.

After all, if we are going to spend so much time depressed then we had better learn how to enjoy it!

Quotes

by un-known

Are they still 'bad habits' if I like them?

The other day I tried an escape room called depression. And I did not escape.

Depression brings people closer to the church, but so do funerals.

The worst part about depression is that people who don't have it just don't get it!

Honestly, I don't even play an active role in my life anymore ...
Things just happen and I'm like "Oh, is this what we're doing now? OK".

In my defence, I was left unsupervised.

I can sympathize with people's pains but not with their pleasures. There is something curiously boring about somebody else's happiness.

That awkward moment when you're wearing Nike's and you can't do it'.

The chains on my mood-swing just snapped... Run.

I wanna be 14 again and ruin my life differently. I have new ideas.

"Sorry, just seeing this now!" Me, to my deep seeded childhood trauma.

Just saying "No" prevents teenage pregnancy the way "Have a nice day!" cures chronic depression.

Satan "Hey, I bought your Soul last month and...!"
Me "No returns!"
Satan "Please it's making me so fucking sad!"

I want someone to look at me the way I look at coffee!"

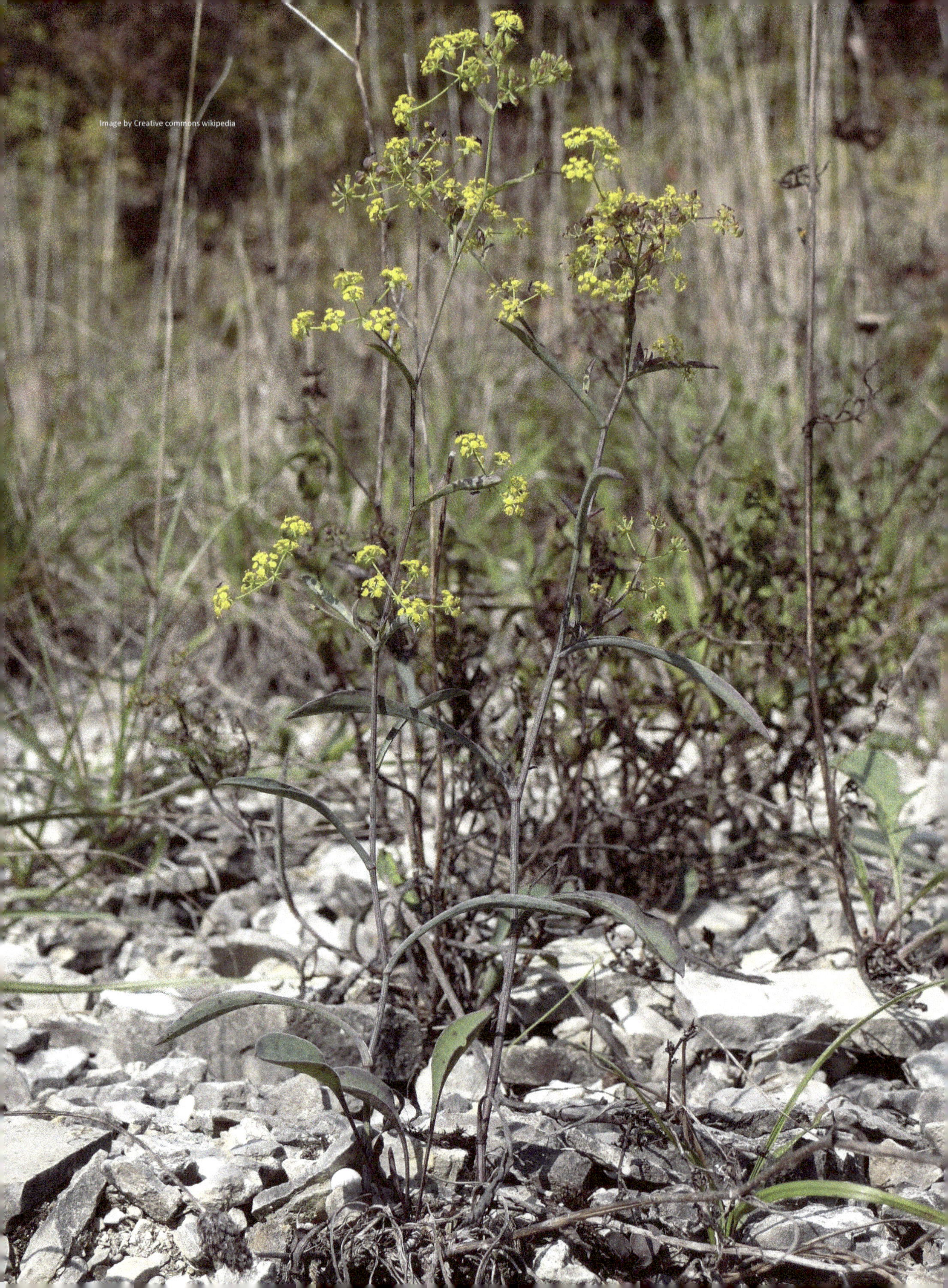
Image by Creative commons wikipedia

Sickle Hare's Ear - Bupleurum falcatum

Bupleurum falcatum is a plain and unassuming herb. However, it has been used for thousands of years in Chinese traditional medicine as a powerful liver tonic and cure for psychosomatic issues. The plant is native to Europe and Western Asia. In more recent times it has been studied for its central nervous system role and subsequent antidepressant actions.

The main compounds attributed to the medicinal effects of the plant are known as saikosaponin-a and -c aglycones, which are primarily found in the roots of the plant. These compounds are thought to be the principal chemicals in the health claims and are known to have immunological, anti-inflammatory, analgesic, anti-allergic and plasma cholesterol lowering effects.

A study conducted in South Korea in 2009 sought to understand the antidepressant action attributed to the herb. In this study, the methanol extract derived from the roots was compared to the standard antidepressant drugs fluoxetine and bupropion. Whilst the two standard pharmaceuticals outperformed the Bupleurum extract, the researchers were able to ascertain a clearer understanding of how the extract worked. Their findings suggest that the extract from the plant influences both the serotonin and noradrenaline levels in the body.

Another report also from South Korea (2018) discussed the anti-inflammatory actions of the herb by regulating immune response activity in the body. Inflammation of the central nervous system is associated with depressive symptoms. Within this report, it was also discussed how the active principle of Bupleurum, saikosaponin, also stimulated nerve growth and retarded amyloid-beta associated plaque build-up on the neurons of the brain.

In 2012, a Chinese paper on the effects of saikosaponins in the treatment of depression was carried out with positive results once again. The researchers used the standard drugs fluoxetine, amitriptyline and paroxetine. Their findings showed that the plant is effective in influencing monoamine function in the prefrontal cortex of the brain. It is this area of the brain that is thought to be involved in depressive related symptoms such as anhedonia (unable to feel pleasure in normally pleasurable activities), and the fear of open spaces and poor diet.

Bupleurum falcatum has also been shown to reduce anxiety and stress. In a trial from Seoul, South Korea in 2011, test animals were subjected to restraint stress, and their responses measured under varying conditions to the levels of stress and anxiety. It was found that at doses of up to 100 mg/kg body weight, a reduction in adrenal stimulation was witnessed and therefore, the researchers assumed that the extract works via the hypothalamic-pituitary-adrenal axis.

Therefore, Bupleurum falcatum reduces stress, anxiety and depression even though it may look unassuming.

[1] R. Article, "Talha Jawaid *, Roli Gupta and Zohaib Ahmed Siddiqui Hygia Institute of Pharmaceutical Education and Research, Lucknow, Uttar Pradesh, India ABSTRACT Depression is a heterogenous mood disorder that has been classified and treated in a variety of ways. A" Int. J. Pharm. Sci. Rev. Res., vol. 2, no. 12, pp. 3051–3060, 2011.

[2] S. Kwon, B. Lee, M. Kim, H. Lee, H. J. Park, and D. H. Hahm, "Antidepressant-like effect of the methanolic extract from Bupleurum falcatum in the tail suspension test," Prog. Neuro-Psychopharmacology Biol. Psychiatry, vol. 34, no. 2, pp. 265–270, 2010.

[3] B. M. Kim, "The role of saikosaponins in therapeutic strategies for age-related diseases," Oxid. Med. Cell. Longev., vol. 2018, 2018.

[4] Xiuping Sun, "Antidepressant-like effects of total saikosaponins of Bupleurum yinchowense in mice," J. Med. Plants Res., vol. 6, no. 26, 2012.

[5] L. Bombi, H. Y. Yun, I. Shim, H. Lee, and D. H. Hahm, "Bupleurum falcatum Prevents Depression and Anxiety-Like Behaviors in Rats Exposed to Repeated Restraint Stress," J. Microbiol. Biotechnol., vol. 22, no. 3, pp. 422–430, 2012.

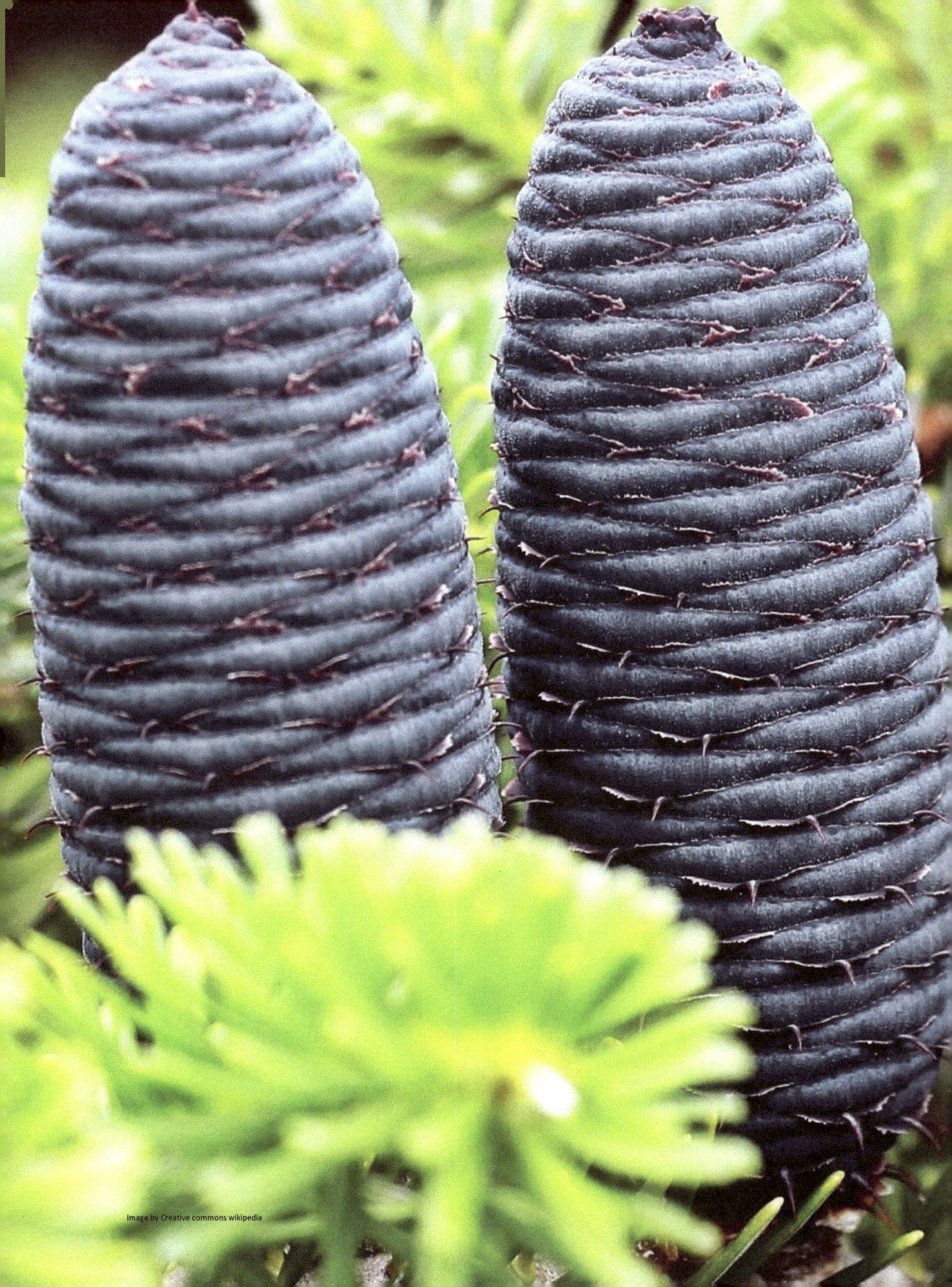
Image by Creative commons wikipedia

Silver Fir - Abies pindrow

Also known as the west Himalayan Fir, the Silver Fir tree grows at high altitudes ranging from 2,000 to 3,300 meters above sea level and spans a territory from Afghanistan to Nepal. The tree is sometimes used as a source of timber, however this is only in localised use as the tree is not grown for commercial timber.

Traditionally, its pine needles or aerial parts have been used as a treatment for anxiety and other nervous disorders by the people living in its native regions. It is nice to imagine that walking through a forest of Abies pindrow was found to be calming, and that therefore someone a long time ago assumed that a cup of tea from the tree's pine needles would have the same effect. Research that trees exhale not only oxygen but all manner of other airborne chemicals, terpenes (volatile oils) make up the essential oil of the tree are some of these exhaled chemicals. Precisely these compounds are thought to be at the core of reason why the plant has calming and relaxing properties. These terpenes are more effectively removed from its needles by an alcohol or methanol extraction process, as it was shown that a water extract of the needles was not very effective in this regard.

Only until recently science studied the tree and its traditional claims in detail. From research conducted in 2015 it was shown that doses of 50 mg per kg bodyweight of the methanol extract derived from the leaves of the tree had anti-anxiety results similar to the standard drug diazepam. Within the research paper it was noticed that extracts made from the tree using water or hexane did not have any effect. This is good news should someone wish to create a new alcoholic beverage for depressive people using the Silver Fir as the base of a new vodka or gin.

A more thorough scientific investigation into the traditional claims of the tree was carried out in 2015. The research focused on a wider range of medical conditions such as depression, anxiety, sleep improvement and anticonvulsant attributes. In all aspects, the methanol and ethanol extract both showed positive results in all of these conditions. In this research the drugs chosen to compare the extracts to were imipramine as well as diazepam. It was shown that doses of 400 mg per kg body weight of Abies pindrow extract was comparable in the mitigation of depression that was achieved by imipramine. The anti-anxiety results were comparable to diazepam. A comforting finding from this research on the antidepressant and anti-anxiety actions of the tree was that the extracts were found to be non-toxic and therefore very safe.

Abies pindrow becomes even more interesting as more recent research in 2016 sought to understand the chemistry found within the tree. To this end these researchers showed that substantial levels of shikimic acid and pinitol exist within the pine needles. Shikimic acid is mainly derived from Star Anise (Illicium verum) and is used as a base chemical in the production of the antiviral medication Tamiflu. Therefore, the use of Abies pindrow may be effective in the treatment of viral infections. However, it has far lower levels of shikimic acid than Star Anise. Pinitol is currently used as a diabetes management drug.

In conclusion, we find Abies pindrow an effective source of anti-depression and anti-anxiety plant extract, and it may be even more useful during the flu season.

[1] D. Kumar and S. Kumar, "Screening of xiety activity of abies pindrow royle aerial parts," Indian J. Pharm. Educ. Res., vol. 49, no. 1, pp. 66–70, 2015.

[2] D. KUMAR and S. KUMAR, "Neuropharmacological Activities of Abies pindrow Aerial Parts in Mice," J. Pharm. Technol. Res. Manag., vol. 3, no. 2, pp. 141–151, 2015.

[3] D. Kumar and S. Kumar, "Quantitative determination of shikimic acid and pinitol in abies pindrow aerial parts using TLC," Indian J. Pharm. Sci., vol. 78, no. 2, pp. 287–290, 2016.

Making medicine

The small scall processing of medical plant material into beneficial products by isolating the medically active parts of the plant is known as galenicals, so named after the 2nd century physician Galen of Pergamon, who became the Roman Empire's greatest physician and is considered the Father of Pharmacy.

There are a relatively small number of methods to prepare the plants. They are, in order of easy to more complicated method of manufacture; infusions/tisanes/teas, decoction, percolation, powder, maceration to extract and tincture, poultice/salve and essential oil.

The basic, general instructions are provided here to indicate how easy it is to manufacture your own, especially as the internet can assist you further. The previous chapter provides a table of plants discussed in these pages and the processes that are suitable for manufacture.

Infusion, tisane (tea)

This category uses water as the solvent or base material, as a general rule.

The processes infusion (and decoction and percolation) are the most basic forms of medicinal production and in remote and isolated communities they represent the easiest and most effective methods of preparation. However, medicines produced by these processes must be used immediately as they have little preservative qualities and may degrade rapidly once made.

The most common form of infusion is simply a tisane. This is where the dried or fresh material is ground coarsely, after which boiling water is poured over it and the preparation is left to stand for some time, usually 15-30 minutes. The water is then strained off and consumed by the patient. One of the most common infusions or tisanes is made from Tea, (*Camellia sinensis*) and is known simply as tea. However, there are many herbal infusions, mistakenly called tea. A recent scientific paper concerning an archaeological dig in China found that tea (*Camellia sinensis*) has been grown and used for over 2,150 years. The name tea comes from the Tang dynasty and is almost directly taken from Northern Chinese language. The terms cha and chai belong to the Southern Chinese languages and they all refer to hot water infusion of the plant *Camellia sinensis*. Therefore, the more appropriate terminology for any botanical infusion is tisane or simply an herbal infusion, and the only tisane that may be called tea is that made from the Camellia plant.

Basic manufacture

Herbal medicinal preparation will require a base or menstruum by which the active ingredients of the plant may be separated and increased. The simplest base is water, yet one of the most popular is ethyl alcohol. Alcohol more easily dissolves the chemistry that is locked in the cellulose of the tree. Other menstruums are methyl alcohol, petroleum, ether and vinegar, to name a few.

The manufacture or distillation of an alcohol base (produces both ethyl and methyl alcohol) is not technically difficult, however it may be open to abuse by the broader community, so knowledge of distillation would require development of professional ethics in medical forestry.

Ethyl alcohol is the most recommended for herbal medicine production due to its ease of manufacture, but also because it is a relatively safe agent, unlike methyl alcohol which can cause serious health problems. Alcohol or ethyl alcohol is easily made from either sugars or starches. The easiest sugar to obtain is cane sugar, sucrose, however it may also be made using fructose from fruit and glucose. The easiest starch source for alcohol production is potato or cassava. The mash, a paste made from potato or other starch vegetable, is mixed with water, and yeast is added. The yeast reacts with the sugars and starches converting them to alcohol. This process takes several days and finishes when no more pressure or bubbling is produced.

After approximately 14 days this first fermenting process will stop. Then distilling will be needed to separate the ethyl alcohol from the wash. In many countries it is possible to purchase a still off the shelf. However, in other countries this is against the law. Yet a still is a simple piece of equipment that can be made from easily obtained materials. In a rural setting all that is required is heat, a pot to heat the wash in, tubing to collect the steam, a condenser to reduce the steam back into a fluid, and a collection pot. The image below shows a simple still.

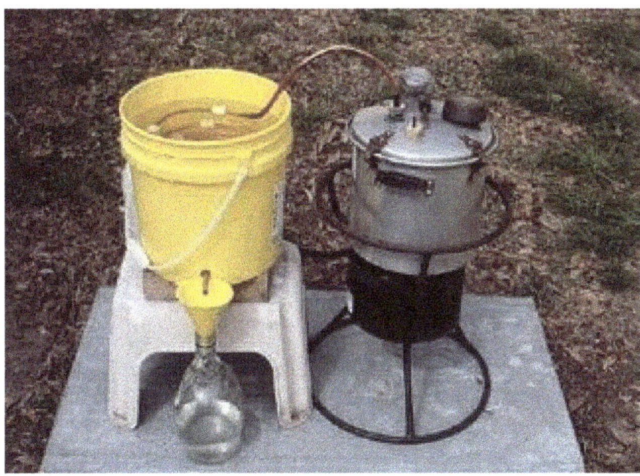

In all methods of producing ethyl alcohol, it must be understood that the first fluid to come out of the condenser in this process will be methyl alcohol and this must be discarded due to health risks. (It leads to blindness and brain damage.) A simple rule is to discard the first 10% of the distilled spirit. This may be difficult to judge due to differing volumes of ethyl alcohol in the wash. Therefore, methyl alcohol turns to steam at approximately 148 degrees Fahrenheit (64.4 Celsius). Once the temperature of the wash in the still passes this temperature and reaches 173 Fahrenheit (78.8 Celsius) the ethyl alcohol will begin to steam and pass through the condenser. Before the temperature reaches approximately 200 Fahrenheit (93.3 Celsius) all the ethyl alcohol should have been passed from the wash to the condenser. At this point no more alcohol will be produced, and the process is finished.

Essential oils

An essential oil is the pure volatile (easily evaporated at normal temperatures) product of a specific plant derived by distillation, or other processes.

The most common method is cold pressing. For example, olives from *Olea europaea* used in the olive oil industry (not volatile), or steam distillation for many medicinal and perfume oils such as those from the lemon tree *Citrus limonum*.

In the alternative, complementary health industry, tinctures, extracts, and essential oils are considered the most effective preparations from plant sources. These essential oils are volatile and do react badly with some containers such as plastics. One great benefit from using essential oils in treating particular health issues is the ability of some to dissolve bacteria. For example, thyme oil (*Thymus vulgaris*) and its active ingredient thymol have been shown to degrade the protein coats of both gram(+) and gram(-) bacteria. In another study a solution of 1% of thyme oil proved fatal to the *Escherichia coli* that causes dysentery. These oils are easily used as they only require simple application to the skin.

This diagram demonstrates that the process of distillation is straight forward and available in remote areas as no electricity is required.

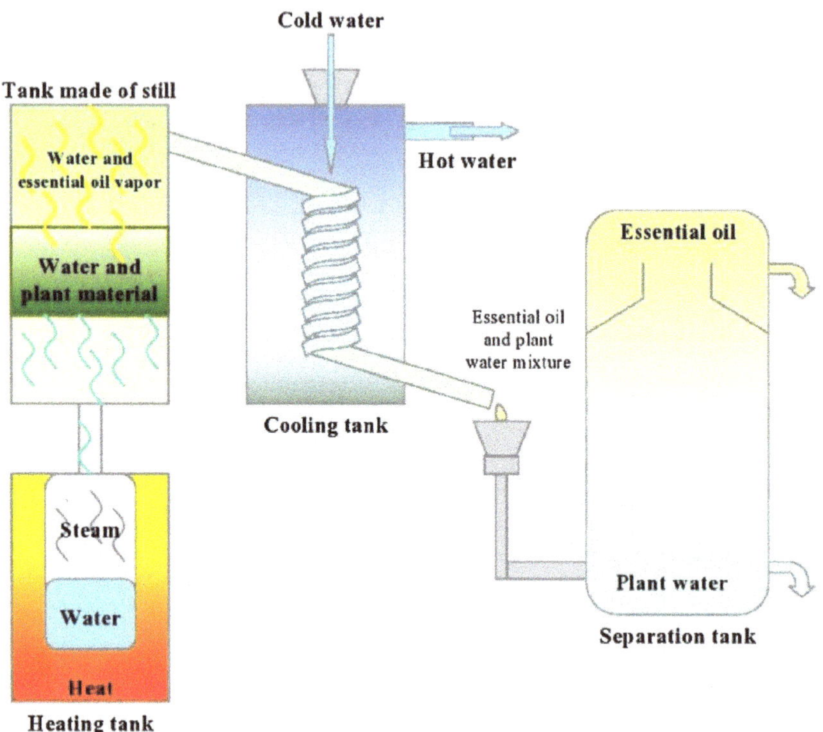

Macerations, Extracts and Tinctures

The process of *maceration* is quite simply, soaking the material in a solvent, menstruum, long enough for the essential ingredients of the material to be transferred into the solvent. Possible solvents are water, alcohol, petroleum and oil. This is the primary technique for making either an extract or a tincture.

The time required for the process to extract all the active parts of plant material will change depending on the type of plant and the different parts of the plant used. For example, the bark of a tree will need more time to macerate than the flowers. The process requires the plant material to be immersed in the solvent until it is exhausted or until nothing further can be extracted. Typically, for simple macerations, three days will be suitable. However, others may take several weeks.

Once the maceration is finished, the solvent is then passed through fine sieves to strain all the remaining solid plant material. These solids are called the *marc*, usually discarded after further pressing to remove any remaining solvent.

While water may be used as a solvent, it is recommended that ethyl alcohol be used when available, as it has a more significant effect on the chemistry of the plant material and therefore extracts much more of the active compounds. Ethyl alcohol is also an extremely effective preservative and will keep herbal preparations in a usable state for a long time. If the patient cannot consume alcohol, for religious or health reasons, then it is a simple process for the herbal extract to be heated to approximately 80 degrees for a reasonable period during which the alcohol will evaporate. This alcohol removal process can be done so that the alcohol is recaptured and is able to be reused. However, heat can damage the benefits in the tincture or extract and reduce the effectiveness of the medicine.

Digestion or Hot Maceration is a variation of the normal maceration process with the addition of gentle heat, especially if hard, woody or thick material is being treated. There are possible adverse effects on the chemistry of the material if the heat is more than approximately 40-45 C degrees.

A Tincture is not as strong as an Extract as it will generally have a 1:5 ratio; that is, only 1 part plant material by weight to 5 parts of solvent by volume. However, tinctures may vary with ratios up to 1:10 with differing ratios of ethanol allowed for in the process, depending on the nature of the plant material and its reaction to ethanol.

In fact, there is a significant level of confusion when discussing Extracts and Tinctures. Often, they are interchangeable, and in some cases, even the Regulatory Body will not differentiate between them (*Therapeutic Goods Administration Australia* 2011). For the purposes of this discussion, it will be assumed that an extract is a medicinal herbal preparation using the maceration process whereby a ratio of 1:1 is achieved, that is, an equal weight of plant material to an equal volume of solvent.

The production of an Extract usually requires a double maceration process or more treatment because the volume of plant material cannot, in most cases, be totally immersed in the corresponding volume of solvent. Only the material that can be totally soaked in the solvent must be used; after it is fully processed, it is then removed from the solvent by filtering and pressing. The used marc is then discarded, and the entire process is repeated with the remaining plant material and the used solvent. In this way, a ratio of 1:1 is achieved.

Alcohol percentages may vary greatly depending on plant material and personal choice. As in any other industry, the Complementary Health Profession has many recipes frequently claimed as intellectual property by practitioners and corporations alike. Most extracts and tinctures will use between 20% and 90% alcohol. The more delicate the plant material, the less alcohol percentage is required. Also, the more oils and resins in the plant material, the higher the alcohol percentage needed. Most preparations have an alcohol content of between 50 – 60%.

Deciphering dosage

To decipher the scientific research in order to arrive at a correct daily dose for treatment is relatively simple and yet of critical importance. In a great majority of the published research papers, the researchers refer to the dry weight of the plant material in doses related to the body weight of the patient.

As an example, in the research paper on *Butea monosperma*, a report from 2016, showed that a dose of 300 mg to 1 kilo body weight of the stem bark from the tree, had slightly lower results in the control of epileptic convulsions as that of the standard drug chlorpromazine. Therefore, the correct dose as cited from the paper for the treatment of epilepsy would be determined by the weight of the patient multiplied by 300 milligrams. The correct dose for a person with a bodyweight of 75 kilograms would be 75 x 300 mg resulting in an amount of 22,500 milligrams dry weight equivalent, per dose, per day.

Yet the type and strength of the liquid extract would also have to be taken into consideration. As discussed, a plant extract may have differing strengths. When the pure, or what may be considered 'prime' extract is to be used of 1:1 (1 part of the plant material to 1 part of the solvent), the calculations are relatively straight forward. A standard ratio for a 1:1 plant extract would be 1 kilogram (kg) of plant material to 1 litre (l) of solvent. At this stage, it would be necessary to convert the 22,500 milligrams (mg) dose into a fluid extract dose. 1 millilitre (ml) of the extract is equal to 1 gram (g) of the plant material, resulting in the need to convert milligrams to grams. This would result in 22.5 grams (g) or 22.5 millilitres (ml) of the extract to be considered equal to the dosage found in the research paper. In a household context, this is slightly more than 4.5 standard teaspoons.

As discussed in the section on extracts and tinctures, the strength of the extract must also be taken into consideration when deciding on the optimal dose. A 1:1 extract ratio was discussed above. Regarding a 1:2 extract ratio, the quantity of solvent would have to be doubled as this extract has 1 part of plant material to 2 parts solvent and is therefore only half as strong as the 1:1 extract ratio.

Again, an extract with a strength of 1:3 has 1 part of the plant material to 3 parts of the solvent and is, therefore, three times weaker than a 1:1 extract.

As another example; researchers found that a leaf extract from a tree has a therapeutic dose at 400 mg/kg body weight. It is being given to a patient with a bodyweight of 82 kg. Therefore, the correct dose when using a 1:1 extract would be:

82 x 400 = 32,800 mg (milligrams)
Converting 32,800 mg = 32.8 grams
Converting 32.8 grams = 32.8 millilitres (ml)
The correct dose, as derived from the research, would be 32.8 ml – per day.

Conversely, the extract may be strengthened or concentrated further by repeating the extraction process with additional herb or plant material in the same solvent or menstruum used before. In this way, an extract may be made with twice or three times the plant material to arrive at a 2:1 or 3:1 extract and as a result, reduce the amount of extract required in each dose. When applying this to the previous example a dose from a 1:1 extract is shown to be 32.8 ml yet in an extract ratio of 2:1 this is reduced to 16.4 ml and a 3:1 extract even further to 8.2 ml dose.

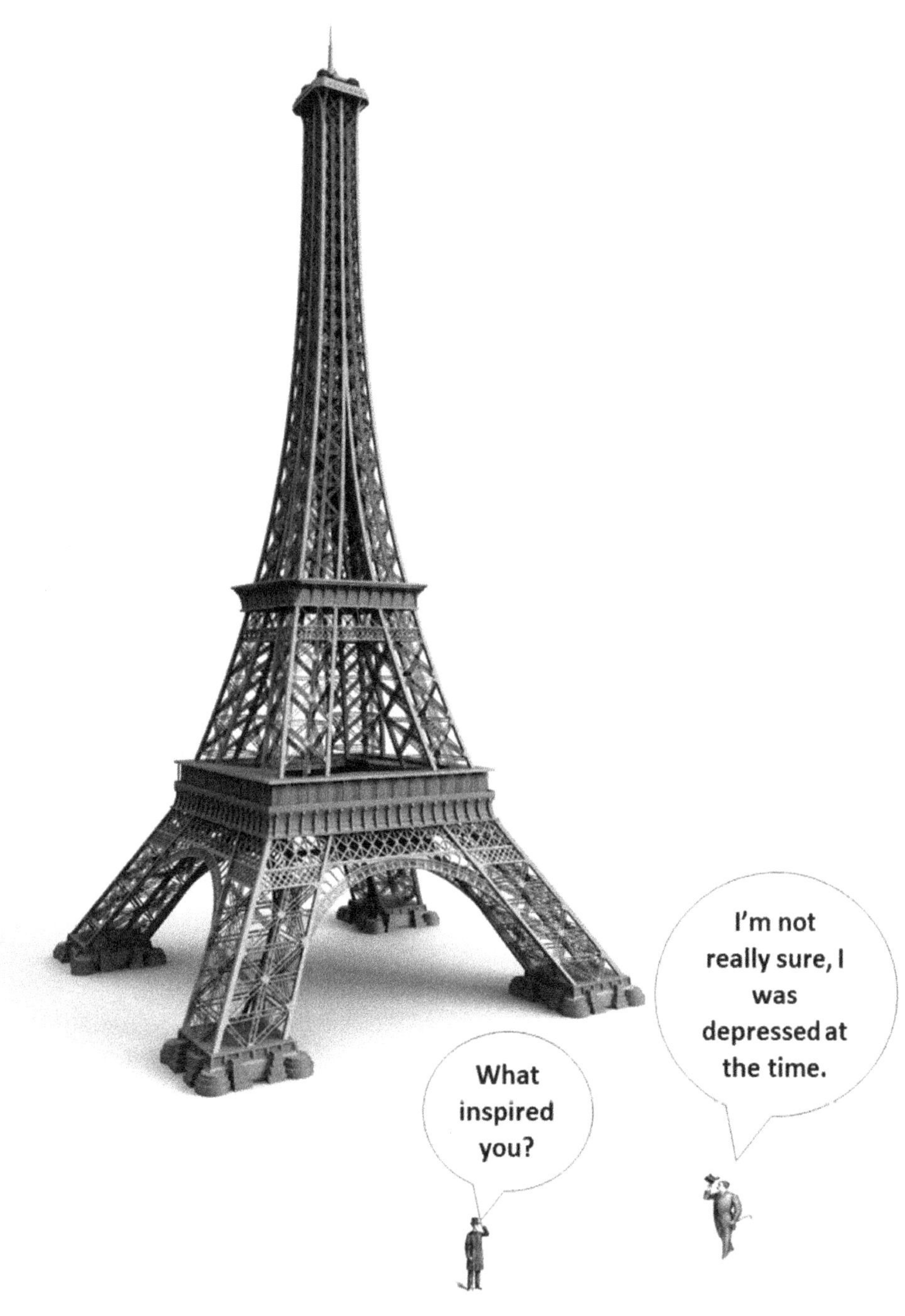
What inspired you?
I'm not really sure, I was depressed at the time.

lticae,

ltice.

スピカナルデイ

セルテイカ

セルテイセ

Spicanardi,

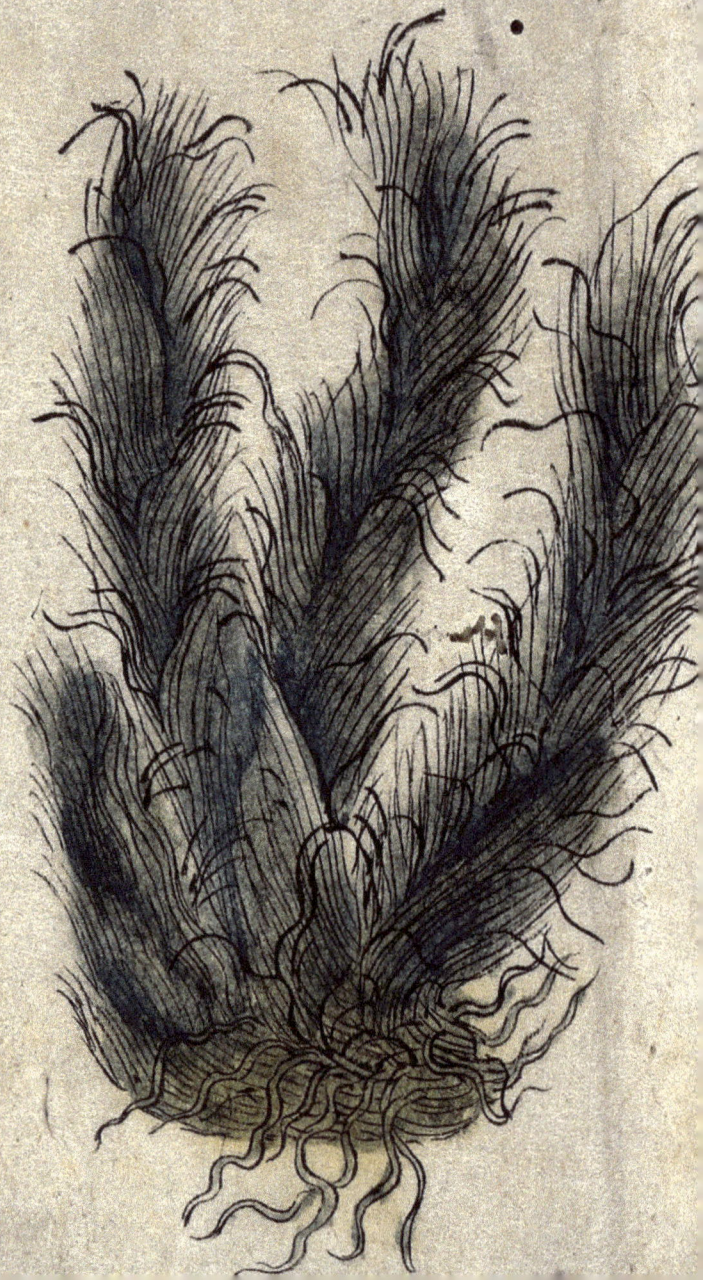

Spikenard - Nardostachys jatamansi

Stepping straight out of an ancient scroll, Spikenard has been revered by the ancient Egyptians and Greeks alike. Originating in the Himalayas, the plant Nardostachys jatamansi grows above 3,000 meters and is now considered critically endangered due to overharvesting. The story of this plant and the oil made from the roots is fascinating and still poorly understood. The trade in the highly priced oil would have required merchants to travel to India, China and Tibet some 3,000 years ago, for the oil to end up in Egypt. The plant is unique to the mountains of Central Asia, and due to its unique climatic requirements, it is very difficult to transplant or cultivate elsewhere.

Several products are made from plants sold as Spikenard, however only the Asian plant N. jatamansi is genuine. The American Spikenard plant is of a different species altogether called Aralia racemose, as is the Japanese Spikenard known as Aralia cordata.

The oil is reported to have an intensely aromatic smell and is amber in colour and viscous. The roots of the plant are distilled to make the oil. In traditional medicine the oil was used as an anti-inflammatory, antibacterial, and to promote sleep. Spikenard has several unique compounds, two of which are named after the plant, Jatamansone and Jatamansic acid.

In 2019, a research paper published in the Journal of Basic & Clinical Pharmacology showed that the ethanol/water extract made from its roots displayed significant antidepressant effects in test animals. The combination of Spikenard extract with the standard drug fluoxetine amplified the potency of fluoxetine and enhanced the antidepressant actions of both. Doses of up to 400 mg/kg body weight were used in the testing.

An early piece of research conducted in 2012 showed that the ethanol/water extract from the roots displayed significant improvement in mice inflicted with radiation-induced depression. This piece of research is fascinating when we consider the amount of radiation surrounding modern lifestyles every minute of the day from microwaves to mobile phones and wireless networks. The Spikenard extract used in this research showed neurological improvements in the test animals. Perhaps Spikenard is more relevant to modern society than it ever was in the ancient world. The researchers used a dose of 200 mg/kg body weight in this testing.

Another study from Iran (2018) sought to understand the mechanism of action on a pharmacological level of N. jatamansi. In this research, the scientists analysed the chemistry within the plant to try and understand how the extract and or the oil of the plant worked in alleviating depression. The Systems Pharmacology Map created from this research supports the use of the plant in treating depression due to its effects on the neurotransmitter activity in the brain.

Another interesting historical fact concerning Spikenard is that the Catholic Church uses the plant in its symbology and states that it signifies Saint Joseph.

[1] A. R. O'Neill, H. K. Badola, P. P. Dhyani, and S. K. Rana, "Integrating ethnobiological knowledge into biodiversity conservation in the Eastern Himalayas," J. Ethnobiol. Ethnomed., vol. 13, no. 1, 2017.

[2] B. Deepa, K. Suchetha, and S. Rao, "Antidepressant activity of nardostachys jatamansi in electron beam irradiated mice," Int. J. Res. Ayurveda Pharm., vol. 4, no. 1, pp. 101–103, 2013.

[3] R. Panchal and N. N. Goswami, "Evaluation of antidepressant activity of hydro-alcoholic extract of rhizomes of Nardostachys jatamansi DC per se and in combination with fluoxetine in wistar albino rats and swiss albino mice," Int. J. Basic Clin. Pharmacol., vol. 9, no. 1, p. 32, 2019.

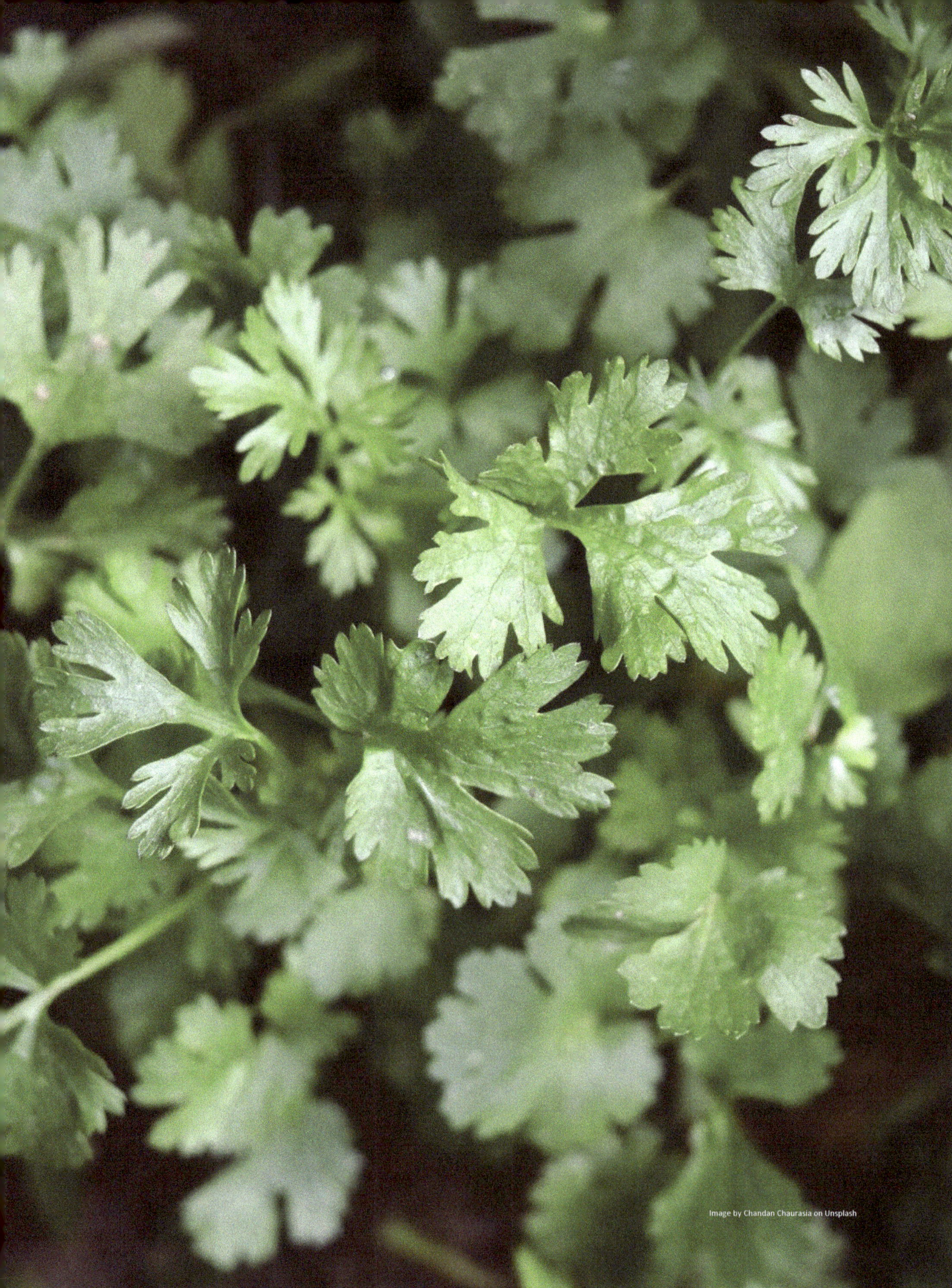
Image by Chandan Chaurasia on Unsplash

Coriander - Coriandrum sativum

Coriander has been found in the archaeological sites of bronze age people as well as in the tomb of Tutankhamen and is now grown all over the world as a spice and green leafy vegetable due to its unique taste. The origin of the plant is thought to be from Iran, however this is still debated due to the confusion created by its ancient use. The Coriander leaves are used as a cuisine ingredient in curries and salads, and the seeds and roots are the most potent part of the plant for medicinal purposes. Interestingly it was listed as one of the original ingredients in the secret recipe for Coca Cola.

The use of this herb must be treated with caution as it has been found that in 32% of children and 23% of adults have an allergic reaction to the plant. So, if you like Coriander in your food, you are probably not allergic to it. However, with these high percentages it is wise to simply wipe some on the sensitive skin under your wrist, and a red inflammation of the skin indicates that you are probably allergic. The ethanol extract from the seeds has been tested for possible toxic effects and at doses of 200 mg/kg body weight no side effects or toxicity was found. So apart from the allergic reactions the herb is considered safe.

A study conducted in Saudi Arabia in 2015 sought to understand the anxiolytic and antidepressant actions of the seed extract. The results of the study showed that the seed extract does have significant anti-anxiety and antidepression actions. They compared the extract to the standard drug imipramine for depression and for anxiety. Whilst the extract was comparable to imipramine for depression, the diazepam outperformed the extract for anxiety. Needless the extract did influence positive outcomes in all the tests. AA dosage of 200 mg/kg body weight was found to be effective.

In an Indian study from 2011 it was shown that doses of 200 mg/kg body weight did outperform diazepam. Therefore, the user must treat clinical research with care as contradictions and competing claims can be confusing at times. So, the researcher must analyse a broad base of research material to try to ascertain the overall outcomes on a weighted average. This is called a Meta-Analysis of Peer Reviewed Papers. Whilst this has not occurred here, another clinical trial from 2015 also agreed that the simple water extract from the leaves of Coriander was similar to diazepam in anxiety and depression models.

The inclusion of the leaves of Coriandrum sativum into a diet has also been shown to reverse memory loss and improve cognitive function of the brain. This function allows us to understand and to relate to the world more effectively. In a study from 2011 a 45 day diet high in Coriander leaf showed significant improvement in memory in test animals in the laboratory. However, the diets consisted of 15% Coriander and as such this may be too much for the average person to bear. Yet, in the extract from this would be far easier. From the same research it was also concluded that the total cholesterol in the brain and also the cholinesterase (an enzyme that retards neurotransmission in the brain) were significantly reduced. Thereby allowing higher functioning of the brain.

[1] A. Pathan, A. Alshahrani, and F. Al-marshad, "Neurological Assessment of Seeds of Coriandrum sativum by Using Antidepressant and Anxiolytic like Activity on Albino Mice," Inven. Impact Ethnopharmacol., vol. 2015, no. 3, pp. 102–105, 2015.

[2] "Anti-anxiety activity of Coriandrum sativum .".

[3] P. Angiosperms, E. Asterids, and A. Apiaceae, "Coriander or cilantro," pp. 1–8, 2018.

[4] "Evaluation of anxiolytic activity of aqueous extract of Coriandrum sativum ."

Index

About the author Paul Evers

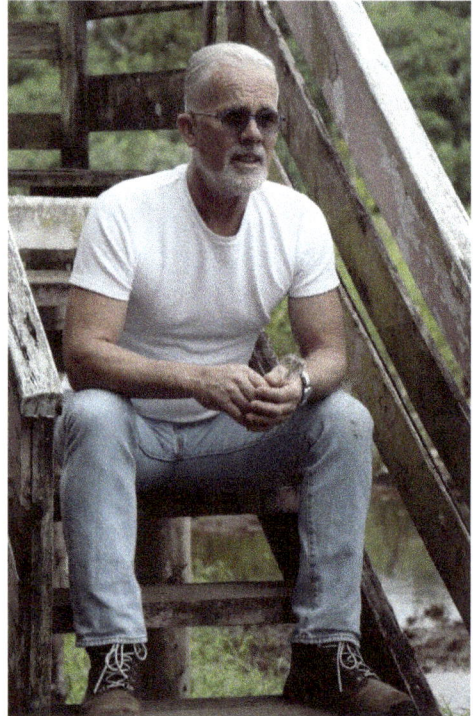

Paul Evers (née Thompson) has his origins in Sydney Australia, as well as the outback of the New South Wales, in the wheat and rice belt in the central west of the state.

In 1988 he gained his qualifications as a naturopath, a practitioner of herbal medicine, from the mother of Australian traditional medicine, Dorothy Hall, who established the Australian Traditional Medicine Society and who published 'Dorothy Hall's Herbal Medicine' that same year.

Years of learning and research commenced with the objective to unleash the hidden medicinal value of growing plants and trees to the benefit of society.

Paul beliefs alternative and traditional medical systems can and must enhance the modern science and technologies of medicine available. He is a longtime advocate of antibiotic restrictions yet is equally a longtime supporter of vaccine therapies.

His unswerving belief is that alternative and traditional medicines must be rigorously researched in order to deliver the best outcomes, especially for almost half the global population who rely on them, whilst at the same time become more integrated in the daily modern medical practices.

The objective of writing about medicinal plants and trees is to elevate the knowledge to a critical asset for population health and wellbeing, and thereby re-connecting humans with their surrounding whilst ensuring the protection of trees and forests into the future.

The challenge in condensing the scientific literature for his books was to arrive at a concise and easily understood review of each plant that excluded un-supported claims.

With more people learning about the health benefits of plants and trees, located close to homes, along roads, in parks, a new and vibrant interest in the cultivation, management and harvesting of these crucial ecosystems can only grow. His books are simply the beginning.

Paul has the gift to connect his research and understanding of the abundant natural properties of plants to the medicinal needs of people, the people surrounding them.

He writes in a conversational tone to reach the general public, to inspire readers to curiosity and discovery.

www.ingramcontent.com/pod-product-compliance
Lightning Source LLC
Chambersburg PA
CBHW041603260326
41914CB00011B/1366

* 9 7 8 0 6 4 5 2 5 1 7 5 3 *